Penguin Books
The Billings Method

D0130002

Dr Evelyn Billings completed her medical degree
at the University of Melbourne and then trained
as a specialist paediatrician. In 1966 she joined her
husband, Dr John Billings, in his research on the
Billings Ovulation Method. Her studies on
breastfeeding mothers and women approaching
the menopause have been a major contribution.
Dr Billings has written numerous articles in scientific
journals and is a co-author of the *Atlas of the Ovulation
Method*. She travels widely each year, teaching and
lecturing about the Billings Method.

Ann Westmore received her scientific training at
the University of Melbourne where she gained a
B.Sc, specializing in physiology and histology.
On graduating, she joined the Melbourne *Sun
News-Pictorial* where she became the medical and
science writer. In 1975 and 1977 she won the
Australian Medical Association's awards for the
best news stories on medical matters. She is now a
freelance journalist, writing mainly about medicine,
science and the environment.

The Billings Method

Dr Evelyn Billings
and Ann Westmore

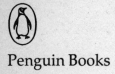

Penguin Books

Penguin Books Ltd, Harmondsworth, Middlesex, England
Penguin Books, 625 Madison Avenue, New York, New York 10022, U.S.A.
Penguin Books Australia Ltd, Ringwood, Victoria, Australia
Penguin Books Canada Ltd, 2801 John Street, Markham, Ontario, Canada L3R 1B4
Penguin Books (N.Z.) Ltd, 182–190 Wairau Road, Auckland 10, New Zealand

First published in Australia by Anne O'Donovan Pty Ltd 1980
First published in Great Britain by Allen Lane 1981
Published in Penguin Books 1982

Made and printed in Great Britain by
Richard Clay (The Chaucer Press) Ltd, Bungay, Suffolk
Set in VIP Palatino

To John

Contents

Acknowledgements

To Dr John Billings, who, responding to the need of couples, recognized the practical value of the cervical mucus as a natural sign of fertility. He showed women how to help themselves by self-knowledge and encouraged them to accept responsibility for it and to teach other women.

To Rev. Fr Maurice Catarinich who by his perseverance and analytical questioning, was responsible for much of the early development of the method. His kind and wise counselling especially in the field of infertility is invaluable.

To the Scientists, especially Professor James B. Brown, who during seventeen years' close association, has provided hormonal monitoring of women's observations of cervical mucus including intensive studies of lactation, pre-menopause and infertility, collaborating with Dr Patricia Harrisson and Dr Meg Smith.

To Professor Henry G. Burger who, working with Professor Brown, established the hormonal correlations with the Peak symptom and the beginning of the fertile phase, thereby producing irrefutable evidence of the validity of the method. He also read the manuscript of the book and offered many helpful criticisms.

To Professor T. Hilgers (USA) for permission to include his research findings and use his illustrations.

To Professor R. Blandau (USA) for the unique photograph from his library.

To Professor E. Odeblad (Sweden) for permission to use his illustrations and include his research findings.

To the many teachers and users of the Ovulation Method who supplied information, illustrations and charts for reproduction; and especially to Dr Kevin Hume, who from his experience both at home and abroad generously offered valuable contributions.

To Mercedes Wilson who devised the stamp system of charting, for the use of her photographs and for her friendly support.

To Ann Westmore who exhibited good humour, patience and skill in her writing of this book, and to Michael her baby son who contributed much to the pleasure of our collaboration.

To Pam Brewster who made charming drawings out of scientific data, very cleverly combining accuracy with beauty.

To Anne O'Donovan whose clear concept of the book was achieved with meticulous care.

EVELYN BILLINGS
1980

1

What is the Billings Ovulation Method?

Throughout history women have sought to control and manage their fertility.

Many primitive methods have been used. In this century, enormous expenditure has been directed towards chemical and mechanical methods of contraception. However, developments such as the Pill, condoms and diaphragms, have their drawbacks. In the case of the Pill the magnitude and severity of its side-effects are becoming increasingly apparent. Many women are turning away from the Pill because of its wide-ranging effects on the body.

Sterilization is widely practised. But many couples find this an unacceptable approach to fertility control.

They see a vacuum, which has *not* been filled by natural methods such as Rhythm and Temperature, methods which have been found to be unreliable and grossly restrictive.

Conscious of this gap, a group of Melbourne doctors and medical researchers has been working on a simple yet substantial discovery: that women themselves can recognize when they are fertile or infertile by the characteristics of the mucus which they can feel and see at the vaginal opening.

The recognition of the importance of the mucus as a marker of fertility is a finding of remarkable significance. For the last twenty-seven years, my colleagues and I have been developing and researching an easily understood, accurate and scientific system of how this dramatic piece of knowledge can be used by any woman.

The basis of the method is awareness of the mucus. This

mucus can indicate whether you are fertile or infertile by its sensation and appearance. It is produced by the cervix, which is the part of the uterus that joins with the vagina, and which is under the control of the reproductive hormones.

It is only in the last decade that the role of the mucus in the miraculous story of human reproduction has been widely recognized. Scientific research has shown that not only does the mucus signal the fertile state, it also appears to be essential if conception is to take place. For without the mucus, sperm transport is impeded and the sperm cells die quickly in the acid environment of the vagina.

When the mucus indicates possible fertility it is necessary to postpone sexual intercourse if a pregnancy is not desired. For most couples, this means that up to half the days of a typical cycle are available for intercourse. In general, days available for intercourse are scattered throughout the cycle so that abstinence is not required for lengthy periods in any cycle. In longer cycles a greater proportion of the cycle is available.

If a couple wants to have a child, the method can help them to achieve this. Indeed, many women experiencing difficulty becoming pregnant have found success by being attentive to the mucus that indicates fertility and timing intercourse to coincide with it.

This method, now known as the Billings or Ovulation Method, is a natural method in that no drugs or devices are needed – just a simple awareness of the changing mucus and the application of this knowledge. It is as effective, properly used, as any other known method of fertility control. The scientific facts are indisputable. The research background to the method is examined in chapter 15. Like some other methods, it is susceptible to the human factor, but couples who are motivated to make it work will find it safe, reliable and simple to use. A few cycles are usually all that is necessary before confidence in the method is assured. A daily record, especially at the beginning, is essential.

Many women have discovered the significance of the mucus themselves, and have used it as a sign of their fertility or infertility even without the scientific verification of the method that is available today. For instance, it is known that at least three African tribal groups (the Taita, Kamba and Luo) have used the mucus produced by the cervix as a marker of fertility for generations past. And an elder of an Australian Aboriginal tribe, Niranji, recently described how young girls of his tribe were taken away to a sacred place by the older women and taught about the mucus.

In western societies, it is not unusual to hear of an individual woman who has discovered for herself the message of the mucus.

The reliability of the method has been demonstrated by a recent World Health Organization one-year trial of the method in five countries (p. 194). Findings indicate an effectiveness of 97 per cent or better. This means that among 100 couples *who follow the method guidelines* for a year, three pregnancies or fewer may be expected to occur. This compares favourably with the effectiveness of contraceptive methods including the Pill and IUD.

The WHO trial results also show that over 90 per cent of women can produce a recognizable chart of their mucus after one cycle.

We know that teaching quality affects the success rate significantly. Most women will be able to learn the method from this book, but some will also find it helpful to consult a trained teacher with whom questions and unusual circumstances can be discussed. A list of the teaching centres is given on p. 200.

What other factors are important in successful use of the method? More than most other methods of fertility control, the method requires a high level of motivation and co-operation.

Couples in a stable relationship usually find it easier to adapt to this method since it requires some days when intercourse should be avoided if a pregnancy is not desired. Successful use calls for partners to act in accordance with the mucus signals of fertility and infertility. This means, for example, that you will need to show your love in ways other than intercourse sometimes.

Natural family planning seems to work best when couples are clear about whether they want to have a child. If they are ambivalent about this, they may test the fertile time and take a chance by deviating from the guidelines.

The method appeals to couples who feel that fertility control is a joint responsibility and that, because of this, neither partner should be required to bear a health burden.

The Billings Method is applicable to all phases of a woman's reproductive life – whether her menstrual cycles are regular or irregular, during adolescence, coming off the Pill, when breastfeeding or approaching the menopause. Each of these special situations is described in a later chapter of the book.

The method causes no side-effects; the natural body processes are not disturbed. This can be an awakening for women who have been using contraceptive medications which alter normal hormone patterns and which can cause irritability, depression, nausea, and sometimes more serious disorders.

Couples are also free of any possible aesthetic objections to using devices such as condoms, diaphragms and IUDs. With this method no equipment is necessary; all the information you need to regulate your fertility comes from your own recognizable mucus pattern.

A bonus of the method is the sense of wonder and deep satisfaction that comes from tuning in to the natural rhythms of your own body.

The method also provides a valuable guide to your gynaecological health. Menstrual cycle irregularities need no longer be a mystery. If an abnormality develops, your mucus will alert you to the problem at an early stage, when treatment is most likely to prove effective.

Women's dissatisfaction with all other known methods of contraception can be heard throughout the world. We have only recently come to realize that Nature herself has provided the answer. The recognition of these fertility signs is like remembering something about ourselves long forgotten.

After reading this book, you will be able to:
- recognize the signs of fertility and infertility
- apply this information and skill to suit your needs
- experience the benefits of the method in terms of satisfaction, happiness, and improved communication with your partner.

2

The mucus discovery

In the 1950s, the only natural family planning method available was the Rhythm Method.

The Rhythm Method is based on the finding that ovulation occurs, on a single day, ten to sixteen days before menstrual bleeding starts. This gives a woman with near regular cycles a means of calculating the days when she is most likely to be fertile. Basing her calculations on the shortest and longest cycles experienced over six to twelve months, she can work out the range of days of possible fertility.

The Rhythm Method is satisfactory as long as cycle length does not change markedly. But it has an inherent fault. No woman is always regular. Inevitably there are significant variations in cycle length – caused by emotional or physical stress, after a pregnancy, or close to the menopause.

The Rhythm Method proved unreliable and needlessly limiting especially when cycles were long and irregular. This is the natural pattern for some women and does not call for corrective treatment unless an underlying abnormality is present. But women with such cycles need to be able to interpret them if they are to be in command of their fertility.

Clearly what was needed was a marker of fertility that women themselves could recognize.

With this in mind, Dr John Billings made a search of the medical literature in 1953. To his surprise – not being a gynaecologist – he found several accounts of a stringy, lubricative mucus, produced at about the time of ovulation by the cells lining the cervix.[1, 2, 3, 4]

Although this mucus had been observed by doctors for

many years, to his knowledge, gynaecologists had never questioned women about their awareness of it.

Indeed, as early as 1855, Smith[5] had stated that conception was most likely to occur when the mucus was 'in its most fluid condition'. Sims[6] in 1868 likewise pointed out the importance of the mucus when he first described the post-coital test for sperm health, saying that it should be carried out when the mucus becomes 'clear and translucent and about the consistency of white of egg'. In 1913, Huhner[7] further investigated Sims's work, and confirmed the desirability of a particular type of mucus for the Huhner's test (described on p. 137). Experiments by Seguy and Simmonet[8] in France in 1933 involving laparotomy, where the ovary is viewed directly, confirmed the time of ovulation and accurately related this to the fertile-type mucus and to the peak of the hormone, oestrogen.

John Billings recognized the possible significance of the mucus as a marker of ovulation. Could the fertile-type mucus be used as a signal of fertility?

After questioning a small number of women, it became clear that the occurrence of different types of mucus during the menstrual cycle was a familiar observation. It then became a matter of determining whether a typical pattern existed during the cycle, and whether women could identify their fertile phase.

With the co-operation of hundreds of women, a standard mucus pattern quickly emerged. It became evident that the sensation produced by the mucus, as well as its appearance, could enable women to recognize the onset of fertility. Even blindness proved to be no barrier to learning. And the pattern appeared similar for women in different societies. (This has been confirmed in the recent five-nation World Health Organization trial.)

My involvement in research and teaching the method began in 1966.

It quickly became clear that woman-to-woman teaching was the most effective way of getting the message across. The basic problem for men who have tried to teach the method is that they can never experience ovulation and therefore only dimly appreciate the observations and sensations of the cervical mucus that provide the key to successful use of the method. Additionally some women find it difficult to talk freely about the mucus to a male teacher.

By the mid-1960s a prolonged clinical study of the mucus had been completed, and a set of guidelines formulated for fertility control.

At this stage, only the mucus pattern associated with ovulation, and the infertile phase following it, had been identified. Rhythm calculations were still used to deal with the first part of the cycle. This was inadequate for women with irregular cycles or delayed ovulation, such as those approaching the menopause or breastfeeding a baby.

However, it became apparent that many women familiar with the method found it unnecessary to take their basal body temperature and were ceasing to do so. They found that the mucus changes alone gave adequate information: that in some women the change from a pattern of dryness to one of mucus signalled fertility; in others a change from a pattern of continuous, unchanging mucus to any mucus that was different, also signalled fertility.

The recognition of the infertile patterns of either dryness or mucus before ovulation, was at the same time a fascinating discovery and a tremendous relief, because it disposed of prolonged abstinence. As long as the mucus or dryness that a woman correctly identified as her infertile pattern remained unchanged, intercourse could not result in conception.

Each step along the way to establishing reliable and universally applicable guidelines for fertility control was tested many times and correlated with hormonal studies.

In 1971, temperature measurements and Rhythm calculations were discontinued. The Billings Ovulation Method, now refined and validated in many studies, could stand alone for all circumstances of reproductive life.

Mothers, knowing whether they were fertile or infertile, could continue to breastfeed their babies. No longer was it considered necessary to wean the baby so that ovulation would occur. Women approaching the menopause could now recognize with confidence their extended phases of infertility, free from anxiety, and the long wait for a rise in temperature that might never occur again.

Opposition to the Ovulation Method came from those who confused it with the Rhythm Method, or who lacked the correct information and expertise to teach it successfully. This opposition stimulated the continued scientific investigations and field trials that have established beyond doubt the validity of the method.

Scientific research into the method initially involved hormonal studies, where a profile of the various hormones involved in reproduction can be obtained from very sensitive measurements. Participants in hormonal studies have included women with normal cycles, nursing mothers, premenopausal women, and those with cycle disorders such as failure of ovulation, disturbed mucus patterns, and women having difficulty conceiving. Investigations of the method have also involved studies of the characteristics of the cervical mucus during the fertile and infertile phases of the cycle. This research has helped many infertile couples with problems of infertility to achieve a pregnancy. In recent years, the techniques of ultrasound and laparoscopy – where the changes occurring on the surface of the ovary can be viewed directly – have been used.

These and other research projects are described in detail in chapter 15, which sets out the scientific basis of the method.

> The laboratory studies of the mucus, the laparoscopic data, the hormonal assays and the infertility research, have all provided confirmatory evidence that a woman's own awareness provides an extremely accurate guide to her state of fertility.

In the following chapters, the practical implications of the mucus discovery are spelt out . . . the 'how', 'when' and 'why' of using the Ovulation Method.

3

Getting to know
your menstrual cycle

The possibility of conceiving a child in any menstrual cycle is limited to a short sequence of fertile days.

This fertile phase is usually about five days in a typical cycle, which averages twenty-three to thirty-five days in length.[1]

Cycles shorter than twenty-three days, and very long cycles of more than thirty-five days, occur from time to time in most women. But the fertile phase remains approximately constant.

Irregular cycles are much more common at the two extremes of reproductive life – adolescence and middle age – than during the years from about twenty to forty. Menstrual irregularities are also common after weaning a baby, or when coming off the Pill.

It is natural for some women to be very irregular and normally fertile. They require no regulating treatment. The Ovulation Method works equally well whether cycles are regular or irregular.

The phases of the menstrual cycle

THE BLEEDING PHASE – MENSTRUATION The number of days of menstrual bleeding in each cycle is commonly four or five, although the reported range is wide. At the beginning of the days of bleeding, which is taken as the start of the menstrual cycle, the ovaries – which are the oval-shaped organs within which the egg cells mature – are at a low level of activity. At this time of the cycle only small amounts of the female

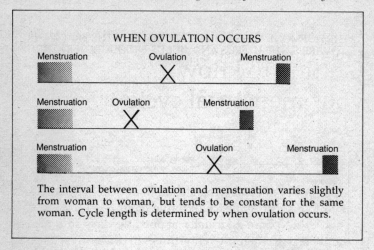

WHEN OVULATION OCCURS

The interval between ovulation and menstruation varies slightly from woman to woman, but tends to be constant for the same woman. Cycle length is determined by when ovulation occurs.

hormones oestrogen and progesterone, are circulating in the blood-stream.

THE PRE-OVULATORY PHASE   As a result of this low-level ovarian activity, the hypothalamus, a walnut-sized collection of highly specialized brain cells, sends out a chemical message, known as a hormone, to the pituitary gland at the base of the brain.

Pituitary hormones which act on the ovaries are triggered. Several nests of cells called follicles, each containing a primitive egg, start to develop within the ovaries, and produce a hormone of the oestrogen group known as oestradiol. This is the hormone which activates the cervix to produce mucus, the substance that appears at the vaginal opening and signals the state of fertility.

Usually only one of the follicles in the ovary reaches full maturity in a cycle. The others, having been active for only a short time, become scar tissue, and they appear to fulfil no further function.

Meanwhile the developing follicle releases larger amounts of the hormone oestradiol, thereby increasing the fertile characteristics of the mucus, while simultaneously moving towards the surface of the ovary. The egg cell within the follicle

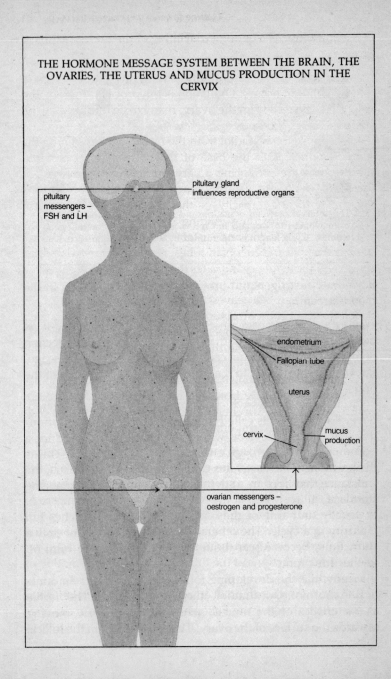

THE HORMONE MESSAGE SYSTEM BETWEEN THE BRAIN, THE OVARIES, THE UTERUS AND MUCUS PRODUCTION IN THE CERVIX

pituitary gland
influences reproductive organs

pituitary
messengers –
FSH and LH

endometrium

Fallopian tube

uterus

cervix

mucus
production

ovarian messengers –
oestrogen and progesterone

is also growing. The endometrial lining of the uterus begins to grow.

OVULATION There is only one day in any particular cycle when ovulation occurs. Ovulation is the process whereby the egg cell is released from the ovary, ready to be fertilized by the sperm.

In response to oestradiol from the ovary, the cells lining the cervix – which is at the base of the uterus and opens into the vagina – are producing a very special type of mucus ... the 'fertile-type' mucus. This mucus is essential in maintaining the fertilizing capacity of the sperm. It enables sperm movement by providing guiding channels and a protective environment for them, and sustains them nutritionally during their journey to the Fallopian tubes. And it captures damaged sperm. All the evidence indicates that unless fertile-type mucus is produced by the cervix, *conception cannot take place*.

When the egg cell leaves the follicle, the remaining cells develop into a yellow structure called the corpus luteum which produces the hormone progesterone, in addition to oestradiol.

These hormones cause the lining of the uterus to further grow and thicken to provide nutrition in preparation for a pregnancy. Progesterone has a profound effect on the characteristics of the mucus from the cervix producing a change which a woman can herself identify. Progesterone also increases the body temperature.

THE POST-OVULATORY PHASE After its release from the ovary, the egg cell has a life-span of only about twelve hours unless it is fertilized by a sperm cell. The numerous finger-like fronds at the wide end of the tube gently sweep the surface of the ovary so that the egg is directed into the tube.

Within its twelve-hour span it starts to move along the funnel-shaped Fallopian tube towards the uterus, aided by wave-like contractions of the tube and the brushing motion of microscopic hairs lining it.

Fertilization – the union of an egg and a sperm – takes place in the outer third of the Fallopian tube, *less than a day after ovulation*.

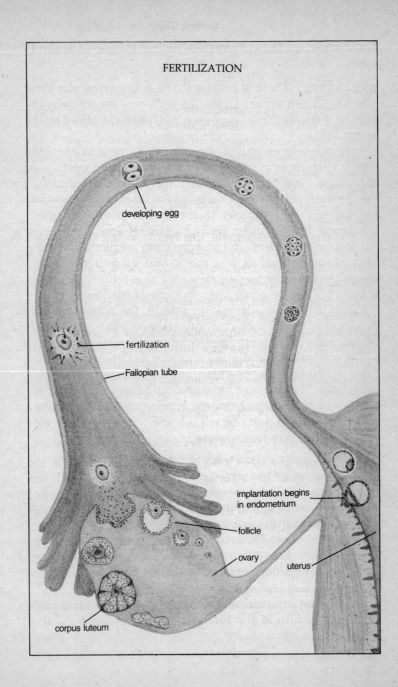

FERTILIZATION

developing egg

fertilization

Fallopian tube

implantation begins
in endometrium

follicle

ovary

uterus

corpus luteum

The final stage of the maturing of the egg does not occur until after fertilization. This fact is reassuring since it demonstrates the vitality of the egg and precludes the development of an old egg.

When the sperm penetrates the outer covering membrane of the egg, its twenty-three chromosomes merge with the twenty-three chromosomes of the egg and a new life (at this stage called a zygote) begins, with a potential life-span of some seventy years. When the sperm and egg fuse, the inherited characteristics of the new individual, such as hair colour, physique, and bio-chemical make-up, are established.

While rapidly developing, this zygote travels along the tube and at about six days begins to embed in the nourishing lining of the uterus, called the endometrium. Implantation is complete by twelve days after ovulation.

The growth of the nutritive endometrium is stimulated by both oestrogen and progesterone, the continued secretion of which is assured by the hormones produced by the implanting zygote. In any cycle, the time during which the endometrium is thickened and filled with nutrients suitable for receiving the developing zygote is only about thirty-six hours. Precise correspondence between stages of development of the fertilized egg and the endometrium is essential for successful implantation.

If the egg is not fertilized it dies and disintegrates. And about fourteen days later (the range is from ten to sixteen days), the endometrium breaks away resulting in menstruation. This shedding of the endometrium occurs when the levels of the hormones oestrogen and progesterone decline.

The process of menstruation has been likened to a tree shedding its leaves in winter: with the next cycle, new growth begins again. New follicles develop, oestrogen is released, and a new endometrium grows in readiness for a possible pregnancy.

Sometimes menstruation occurs without the release of an egg cell. The cycle is then termed anovular. Such cycles are more common around the time of puberty or at the menopause, when hormone levels are insufficient to cause the egg to be released.

However, under the influence of oestrogen, the lining of the uterus still grows, and is shed in the form of menstrual bleeding when the level of the hormone declines.

Other changes during the menstrual cycle

The hormonal events of the menstrual cycle cause psychological as well as physical changes which vary from woman to woman. Most women are aware of altered moods and physical characteristics corresponding to different stages of their cycle. Emotional peaks and troughs both immediately before and during menstruation have been documented, ranging from irritability, depression, anxiety and fatigue, to elevated mood states.

It is common for breast tenderness and lumpiness to precede menstruation, and this may cause feelings of discomfort. Some women report migraine headaches during the first day or two of bleeding. Lower abdominal pains bear a variable relationship to ovulation.

Around the time of ovulation, the mucus at the vaginal opening undergoes significant changes. The mucus – produced by the cervix – provides the key to recognizing your fertility. It will be discussed in more detail in the next chapter.

By developing an awareness of the events of the menstrual cycle and especially the changes in the mucus, women can learn to recognize their fertility or infertility with precision.

4

The key to fertility control – the mucus

When the ground is dry a seed will not germinate. But when the rains come prepare for a harvest. So it is with a woman, that when she is wet with the mucus and for three days afterwards she may expect the harvest of a baby.
– Teaching the Ovulation Method in the World Health Organization study, El Salvador, central America

We usually represent the menstrual cycle as beginning with the menstrual bleeding and ending as the next period of bleeding starts. In a fertile cycle, you ovulate on one day only. Even when two eggs develop (as happens with twins) both are released on the same day. If no pregnancy occurs, your menstrual bleeding will start about two weeks after ovulation.

The sensation of wetness associated with menstruation is often your first indication of a period. So it is with fertile-type mucus . . .

Sometimes during your cycle you wonder if a period has started. You feel something wet and slippery outside the vagina. When you check, you see a white, or clear, stretchy mucus. You may think – 'Oh well, that's nothing.' But far from being nothing, this mucus – the fertile mucus – is a most important sign of good health and fertility. It is produced by the cells of the cervix for an average of six days before ovulation.[1]

The fertile-type mucus appears to be essential for fertility. Both clinical and laboratory studies have shown that the most fertile time in the cycle coincides with the fertile-type mucus, and that infertility is associated with absence of the fertile-type mucus in otherwise normal women.

This mucus provides the sperm cells with a protective envelope so that the sperm retain their fertilizing capacity for three days, and occasionally for as long as five days (but only if mucus is present). Without it, sperm cells deteriorate rapidly: even minutes in the normally acid environment of the vagina will cripple sperm.[2]

The fertile-type mucus nourishes the sperm cells by supplementing their energy requirements and in some way not yet fully understood, may make the sperm cells capable of fertilizing the egg. The mucus acts as a filter, destroying damaged sperm cells. Every ejaculate contains a proportion of these.

As well as providing protection and nourishment, the mucus also forms guiding channels which help the sperm to move along the vagina, through the cervix and uterus, and into the Fallopian tubes. Even mucus outside the vagina can enable sperm cells to reach the egg. (Thus pregnancy can result following genital contact without full penetration taking place.)

While learning to recognize the types of mucus that indicate fertility or infertility, it is important to keep a daily record of your observations.

Do not be concerned that your pattern does not conform to that of other women. Episodes of fertile-type mucus may be longer or shorter in duration and, in quantity, the mucus may be more or less. Each woman will find that she has her own recognizable pattern which is as individual as she is.

Watch for changes in the sensation and appearance of the mucus. These are the vital indicators of altered fertility.

Most women quickly grasp the pattern of their fertility, but a trained teacher will ensure that you are correctly interpreting

THE SPERM AND THE MUCUS

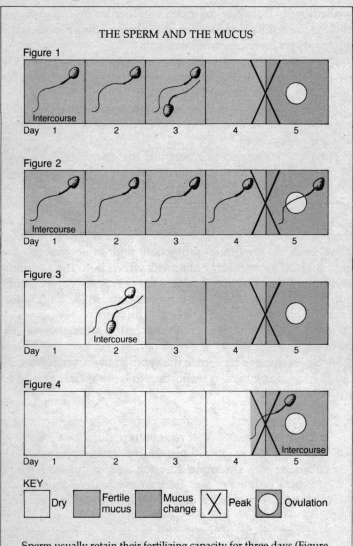

Sperm usually retain their fertilizing capacity for three days (Figure 1), but under optimal mucus conditions, occasionally for up to five days (Figure 2). If intercourse takes place on a dry day (Figure 3), sperm fertilizing capacity is quickly impaired. If intercourse occurs on or just after the Peak (Figure 4), conception is most likely.

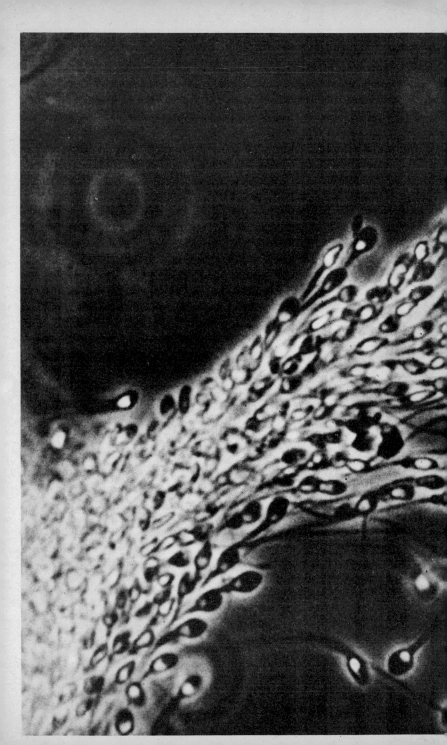

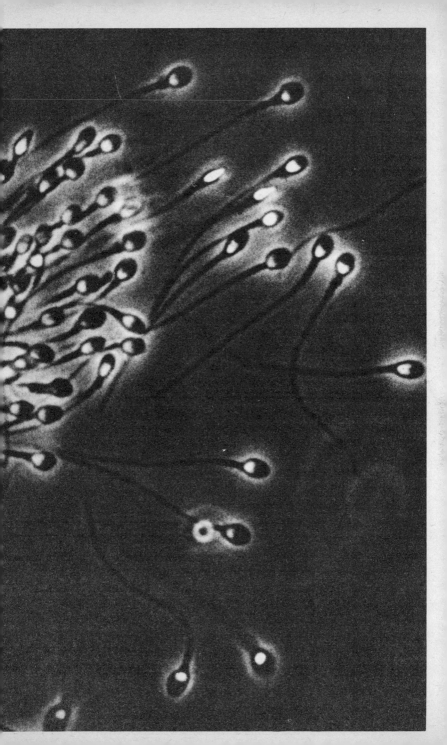

your record. It may also help to talk to other women who are using the method.

While learning the method it is necessary to avoid inter-course during the first month of recording. This enables you to gain a clear picture of your mucus pattern. It is possible for seminal fluid or vaginal secretions associated with intercourse to confuse the picture while you are getting to know your mucus pattern.

What sort of pattern can you expect?

The Basic Infertile Pattern (BIP)

In one common type of cycle, the sensation you experience after your menstrual bleeding is dryness. No mucus is seen or felt, and this is described as a *Basic Infertile Pattern of dryness*.

In the other common pattern, there are no dry days after menstruation. Mucus is visible, and it is usually dense, flaky, and scant in amount. It may produce a sensation of stickiness. And it continues day after day *without change of any kind*. This unchanging mucus is described as a *Basic Infertile Pattern of mucus*.

In a typical twenty-eight day cycle, a BIP of dryness or of mucus lasts for two to three days after the menstrual bleeding.

While dry days can be determined during the first month of charting, several cycles may be necessary to interpret with confidence the BIP of mucus, and the point of change to fertile-type mucus.

The fertile-type mucus

The first indication of the change leading to ovulation may be sticky thread-like mucus after dry days, or a feeling of moist-ness after a succession of sticky days.

These sensations are experienced on the skin outside the

The photograph on the previous pages shows sperm moving through the fertile mucus (*Dr R. Blandau*) vagina. You may see a lump of cloudy mucus that has been resting like a plug in the cervix. As the days pass, you will notice that the mucus becomes thinner, clearer, stringy, and more profuse.

Women use all sorts of expressions to describe this fertile-type mucus . . . looping, like strings of raw egg-white, smooth or slippery.

It may be clear, cloudy, or tinged with blood in which case it may look slightly pink, brown, red or yellow.

This fertile mucus will always have a wet, slippery property because of its chemical structure and composition.

A characteristic odour of the fertile mucus is familiar to many women. This has been noted particularly by the blind.

The fertile phase begins, with a change from the BIP, on average six days before ovulation.

For however many days the mucus is present, it provides ample warning of the approach of ovulation and the need for absolute avoidance of intercourse and genital contact if a pregnancy is not desired . . . for sperm are kept alive and healthy by this fertile-type mucus.

The sensation and appearance of the fertile-type mucus may be accompanied by a feeling of fullness, softness, or swelling in the tissues around the opening of the vagina. It's like a ripening – something which many women can associate clearly with fertility. No other signs of fertility, such as pain or spots of blood, are as precise or reliable as the mucus.

When the general vaginal region is lubricated by this fertile mucus, libido and interest in lovemaking may be heightened. Mistakenly, some women think that sexual desire produces the secretion.

The Peak of fertility

The last day of any of the fertile characteristics of the mucus – that is, the last day when it looks stringy or stretchy or produces a sensation of lubrication, is the *most fertile day* of the cycle.

You will know it is the last day only in retrospect. This day is called the Peak of fertility, because it is the day when intercourse is most likely to result in a pregnancy. It is important to realize that it is not necessarily the day of *most mucus*. This is a common error.

The key to the Peak is that it is the *last day of any of the fertile mucus characteristics* – that is, the last day when the mucus at the vaginal opening looks stringy or feels lubricative. The lubricative sensation may last a day or two longer than the appearance of strings of mucus, indicating that you are still highly fertile. The sensation is the most valuable sign. Some women will see no mucus.

Studies show that the Peak mucus signal usually occurs within a day of ovulation (p. 179).

Over 90 per cent of women can identify the fertile phase and the Peak day of fertility in the first month of observation (World Health Organization trial, p. 195). Encouragement and practice can further increase this figure. The occurrence of a menstrual period approximately two weeks after your estimated Peak will confirm your observations and your confidence will grow with succeeding cycles.

The small number of women who cannot identify a recognizable mucus pattern require special assistance; they may need to be particularly alert to the sensation that the mucus produces outside the vagina. Sometimes only a small amount of mucus is produced and sensation will be the prime guide. This is important for a woman having difficulty conceiving.

A few women will find it difficult at first to believe that reliable signs of fertility are available and will think they have no mucus. They may have dismissed any chance observations of wetness as due to intercourse or stimulation, or even to infection.

Do not be discouraged. By being alert to the changing sensations that even a minute quantity of mucus produces, you will soon learn your own signs of fertility.

If you are having difficulty in determining your fertile phase, daily temperature measurements for a few cycles may prove helpful in indicating whether you are ovulating or not.

THE FEMALE REPRODUCTIVE SYSTEM SHOWING THE EFFECT OF THE MUCUS ON SPERM MOVEMENT

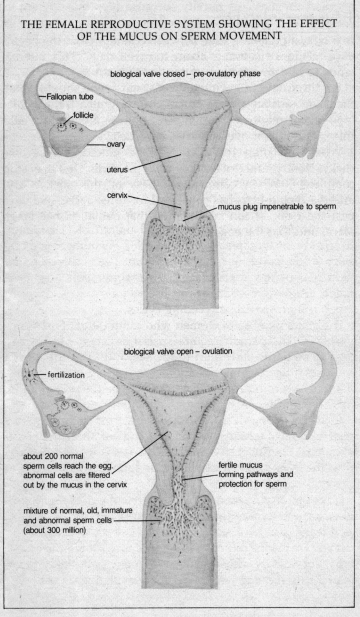

biological valve closed – pre-ovulatory phase

Fallopian tube

follicle

ovary

uterus

cervix

mucus plug impenetrable to sperm

biological valve open – ovulation

fertilization

about 200 normal sperm cells reach the egg. abnormal cells are filtered out by the mucus in the cervix

fertile mucus forming pathways and protection for sperm

mixture of normal, old, immature and abnormal sperm cells (about 300 million)

The post-ovulatory phase

In a typical cycle, the time between ovulation and the beginning of menstruation is about fourteen days. This interval tends to remain constant for the individual.

For three days following the Peak signal, you should watch the characteristics of your mucus very carefully. If the fertile-type mucus reappears within three days of a doubtful Peak, this suggests that ovulation has been delayed.

When ovulation has occurred, the mucus will become sticky, cloudy, and dry for the rest of the cycle. Or it may stop completely. When complete dryness or this sticky, dry, infertile-type mucus has continued for three successive days past the Peak, it can be assumed that ovulation has taken place, and that the egg cell is dead.

5

Keeping your mucus record

The most effective way of learning to recognize your mucus signals is to record your observations daily on a chart. The aim is to identify on any day whether intercourse could or could not result in pregnancy. You will be ready to use the method after observing for one month.

For quick, easy reference, a set of coloured markers has been devised to record observations. At first, observations are made using only red, green and white stamps. These are interpreted by study for a cycle or two. After this learning stage the mucus patterns can be identified and recorded as infertile or possibly fertile. Always observations, not interpretations, are recorded.

Keeping a record of your mucus becomes second nature. It merely requires that you attach the appropriate sticker to the chart every evening, and add a few words to describe the sensation produced by the mucus outside the vagina, and its appearance, during the day. Charts and stamps are available from the centres listed on p. 200. If you are unable to obtain these, you may wish to devise your own chart using coloured pencils.

Several different systems of recording cycles have been invented. Buttons of different shapes are strung on a string by the blind. Teachers in developing countries have adapted the method to meet the needs of the local community. Women in some parts of India tie knots in a rope looped around the waist, while in other countries information is scratched on the trunk of a tree. Women in Papua New Guinea thread coloured beads on a string.

Daily recordings help you to become familiar with your mucus patterns in normal cycles; when stress delays ovulation; and in altered reproductive circumstances – such as when a pregnancy is desired, or during breastfeeding, or when approaching the menopause. Typical examples of charts while learning the method, and for long and short cycles, are illustrated in Figures 1, 2 and 3 (p. 114).

OVULATION METHOD COLOUR CODE

RED for days of bleeding or spotting.

GREEN when no mucus is observed and there is a sensation of dryness.

WHITE for mucus that is possibly fertile.

YELLOW for infertile mucus i.e. mucus that remains the same day after day after day. Infertile mucus can only be recognized as such after studying a cycle or two. Thereafter, the yellow stamp means possible fertility. Distinction between infertile and possibly fertile mucus is necessary when mucus occurs frequently before ovulation. Yellow stamps are also used for mucus after ovulation. These days are infertile because the egg is dead.

The first and most important step in learning the method is to develop an awareness of the mucus and its changes.

If your mucus signs are unclear, it may be helpful to discuss them with an Ovulation Method teacher. There are now many such teachers throughout the world. For information write to your Ovulation Method Centre.

If you are ovulating rarely, for instance while approaching the menopause, or if you have not ovulated since the birth of a child, you can learn to recognize your Basic Infertile Pattern after keeping a chart for about two weeks. *Any change from this pattern signals a possible return of fertility.*

During the initial month while learning to assess your mucus signals through charting, it is recommended that you do not have intercourse and avoid all genital contact, including withdrawal. Barrier contraceptive devices, such as condoms or diaphragms, should not be used, for the pattern of cervical mucus may be obscured by seminal fluid or vaginal secretions released during sexual activity.

Many women discontinue daily charting when they are confident of their ability to interpret their mucus accurately. However it is advisable to continue to keep a record of your mucus, if there is a serious reason to avoid pregnancy.

How do you observe the mucus?

SENSATION The mucus produces a sensation on the skin outside the vagina. This is the more important observation. As you go about your normal activities you may be aware of a sensation of wetness, stickiness or of nothing at all (dryness).

Even a very small non-visible quantity of mucus can change the sensation from dry to not-so-dry, sticky, moist, slippery, or wet. Some women will be discouraged if they expect to *see* mucus which looks like clear raw egg-white and which stretches without breaking.

APPEARANCE At any time you feel the presence of the mucus you can note its appearance. Women have their own individual ways of doing this. Some women pass a tissue across the vaginal opening before passing water. A woman learns to evaluate her own observations which are personal to her. A consistent routine of making observations is recommended.

If there is sufficient mucus to be seen and collected, it can then be checked for clarity, stretchiness, blood staining, thickening, colour changes, stickiness, glueyness, blobs and lumps and changes in quantity.

The fluidity of highly fertile mucus causes it to stretch easily and ensures its presence outside the vagina very soon after its production in the cervix. You do not need to examine the inside of the vagina. It is always moist, and thus confusion is likely to result.

Very tight undergarments, such as pantygirdles, sometimes

make it difficult to feel the sensations outside the vagina. Since these sensations are extremely important indicators of your state of fertility, it is preferable to wear underclothes that are sufficiently loose to enable you to tune in to your sensations.

When do you check the mucus?

There is no particular time of the day. Most women using the method automatically make a mental note of any mucus when they go to the toilet. They are also alert for sensations around the vaginal opening at any time.

Use your own words when, at the end of every day, you note down the sensations and appearance of the mucus, particularly the most fertile sign that you have experienced during the day.

Your description need not mean anything to others. Simply record your mucus observations without trying to interpret them at first. Women who say that they neither feel nor see any mucus are often surprised at what they notice once given basic information about what to look for. They often produce a classic pattern at the first attempt.

In a new situation, such as when breastfeeding or approaching the menopause, it is advisable to resume charting. In such circumstances, infertility may be the dominant state and Peaks of fertility may occur only occasionally or not at all; *recognition of infertility* is now the key to controlling your fertility.

One important bonus of keeping a chart for some couples is that it may open up areas of discussion about intimate and vital matters including fertility regulation. For the method demands communication about emotions and sexuality, and this often enhances a relationship.

Some men like to see the chart so that they can accommodate themselves to its requirements. For instance, they will know whether it is desirable or undesirable to have intercourse at a particular time of the cycle, if the intention is to avoid a pregnancy. In this way, they can give support and assurance to their partners about following the guidelines.

This joint approach to fertility control is in line with the growing awareness that the combined fertility of both partners at any particular time determines whether or not a pregnancy occurs. The sharing of responsibility for a pregnancy lifts the burden of fertility control from one partner, and encourages an attitude of mutual and responsible loving that is the foundation of successful and intelligent family planning.

When are you fertile?

The length of the fertile phase depends on the combined fertility of yourself and your partner.

That is, it depends on the rapid transport and maintenance of the fertilizing capacity of the sperm (typically two or three days and occasionally up to five days) – which is directly related to the presence of fertile cervical mucus – as well as the time of release of the egg and its subsequent survival (typically the egg lives for about twelve hours).

For the average couple, the time during which conception may result from intercourse in a cycle of any length is three to six days.

This may extend to seven days in highly fertile couples. In other couples it may be only half a day, due to the short duration of the presence of the mucus, and this short fertile phase may occur in occasional cycles only.

The guidelines described in the next chapter provide a built-in safety margin to minimize the possibility of an unplanned pregnancy.

6

Applying the method– the guidelines

In these guidelines, abstinence from intercourse includes the avoidance of all genital contact. This is because healthy sperm cells can move from outside the vagina to the Fallopian tubes when fertile-type mucus is present. In this way an unintended pregnancy may occur.

When intercourse is inadvisable, don't give up loving altogether.

'We have found a limitless set of possibilities in our sexual relationship, since using the Ovulation Method. Sexuality is loving, understanding, touching, being close, and exploring a vast range of shared experiences.'

Guidelines to avoid a pregnancy

THE EARLY INFERTILE DAYS – THE EARLY DAY RULES
The early infertile days are the days before any change occurs. These days may be dry, without any sign of mucus; or you may have mucus which, be it flaky, sticky or dense, remains the same day after day after day.

Both these patterns are referred to as a Basic Infertile Pattern (BIP) – the first is a BIP of dryness; the second a BIP of unchanging mucus. Both indicate that you are infertile. A *change* in either case indicates possible fertility.

Intercourse should be confined to the evenings in the early part of the cycle so that the Basic Infertile Pattern can be confirmed during the day. Otherwise a change to the fertile-type mucus may occur during the night, and you and your partner – unaware of your increasing fertility – may have intercourse in the morning which could carry some possibility of a pregnancy.

Intercourse on alternate days will provide greater safety, because seminal fluid and vaginal secretions tend to obscure the mucus on the day following intercourse. Twenty-four hours is sufficient for the seminal fluid to disappear completely.

If your BIP is dry days, and these are interrupted by a day of mucus, it is advisable to avoid intercourse on this day and for three days afterwards. This three-day margin allows the pattern to become either possibly fertile or obviously infertile. If the BIP of dryness returns without recognition of the Peak, once again alternate evenings are available for intercourse.

If the BIP is days of continuous, unchanging mucus, and this is interrupted by a day when the mucus has changed, once again, avoid intercourse on this day and for three days afterwards. If your BIP of mucus returns, you may safely have intercourse on alternate evenings. The BIP occurs before ovulation only.

FERTILE DAYS – THE PEAK DAY RULE   Any *change* in the amount, colour, consistency, stringiness or wetness of the mucus indicates some activity in the ovaries, and the possibility that you are fertile.

Abstinence from intercourse should begin as soon as any change from your BIP is observed or felt. Continue to avoid intercourse during the days of fertile-type mucus and for three days after the last day of any fertile sign. The last day of a sensation of lubricativeness or the appearance of any clear or stringy mucus, is known as the day of Peak fertility. It coincides closely with ovulation. (See chapter 15.)

THE LATE INFERTILE DAYS   The late infertile days begin on the fourth day after your Peak (that is, after you have recognized the Peak and avoided intercourse for the next three days) and continue until the end of your cycle. They are the days when the combined fertility of you and your partner is zero.

Ovulation is over and the egg is dead. Once the Peak has been identified correctly no abstinence is required beyond the third day. Intercourse at any time of the day or night carries no possibility of a pregnancy.

DURING MENSTRUAL BLEEDING Couples should defer intercourse during these days. This ensures that ovulatory signs are not obscured by the bleeding. During a short cycle, ovulation may occur before the bleeding has stopped; and the advice to avoid intercourse at this time takes account of this.

DURING ANY DAY OF BLEEDING BEFORE THE MENSTRUAL PERIOD Avoid intercourse then, and for three days after the appearance of any spots of blood. For such bleeding may coincide with ovulation, and tinge the slippery stretchy mucus pink, brown, red, or yellow. Correct mucus identification is difficult if the bleeding is heavy.

STRESS SITUATIONS Anxiety, stress, travel, illness, or change of environment may delay or abolish ovulation in a cycle even after the chain of events leading to the release of the egg is in motion. If you experience severe stress, for example, you should anticipate the possibility of delayed ovulation, and take special care in evaluating the Peak of fertility. Delaying intercourse in the event of a confused pattern due to stress is a sensible approach.

'My reason for using the method is that I definitely do not want any more children at the present time. I find my capacity to look after my loved three children already strained to the utmost.

I feel that if anyone wants to use the method for this reason, they really need to go into it very thoroughly, and not cut any corners or take risks with it.

At first my husband and I found it very limiting, and certainly not all sweetness and light. Not being able to have intercourse at certain times is a situation that needs to be fully shared and accepted by both partners. As time went on however, we found this aspect less frustrating; we found we were becoming more aware of each other's needs and feelings. I feel that for us, it has caused a development in our relationship and a deepening of our love.

It is four years since Dr Lyn Billings explained the method to me, and I feel that I am now in a far better position to cope with our family situation, and that the life in this family is far more peaceful and stable. (Of course, other factors come into this also.)

I would also like to make the point that before I began using the method, I had been on the Pill for twelve months. I did not like being on the Pill at all, and really felt more like a 'thing' than a person. I did not like using chemicals which I knew could have side-effects – and far prefer to know at what stage of the normal cycle I am.'

Guidelines to achieve a pregnancy

Aim to have intercourse two or three times a week before the fertile signs appear, while maintaining a close check on your mucus pattern so that you can detect signs of fertility.

If you usually have several days of fertile mucus in a cycle, aim to have intercourse on these days, as close to the Peak as possible.

If you produce fertile-type mucus only in some cycles, and for only a short time during the cycle, have intercourse at this time. Precision is extremely important for conception. Mucus present for only part of a day is, in some women, sufficient for conception to occur.

7

Questions often asked

Is the Billings Ovulation Method more suitable for some couples than others?

Yes, couples in a stable relationship usually find it easier to accept a method that requires some days without intercourse.

The method requires commitment. It appeals most strongly to couples who are motivated to use a natural method and who are willing to take joint responsibility for fertility control.

The method is most suitable for a man and woman who love each other. It helps to generate love. In the absence of loving concern, it will not work.

How do I know when I am fertile?

Your cervical mucus will indicate whether you are fertile or infertile by its characteristics:
• A sensation of dryness, with no mucus, indicates infertility.
• Mucus which is flaky, opaque, sticky, and scant, and which continues without change day after day also indicates infertility.
• Mucus which differs from either of these patterns suggests an altered level of fertility. If the mucus feels slippery and wet, looks like raw egg-white and can be stretched to form a delicate thread before breaking, you are probably at your most fertile time.

Keeping a daily record will show how the mucus changes from time to time. *The pattern of behaviour of the mucus* is the best way to recognize both fertility and infertility rather than an initial judgement about any particular type of mucus. Every woman's mucus pattern is a little different, but she quickly learns to recognize it herself.

How do I find the mucus?

You will find the mucus at your vaginal opening. You do not need to feel inside the vagina; this will merely confuse the picture because the vagina is always moist. Check for the mucus routinely during the course of the day. Be alert to the sensation it produces, as well as to its appearance. Tuning in to your fertility will soon become second nature to you.

Do I need to keep a chart of my mucus pattern?

Most women find that some sort of recording is necessary as they learn to recognize the different types of mucus associated with fertility or infertility. Don't rely on your memory.

A chart can prove helpful to your partner in giving him an understanding of the mucus changes and communicating your state of fertility. For the purposes of learning, it is advisable to keep a chart for a few months.

Once you are confident that you can recognize your mucus pattern, you can continue with the chart or merely turn your attention to the sensation and appearance of your mucus when you want to know your state of fertility. It is advisable to continue charting if you have a serious reason to avoid pregnancy; or while in a situation of altered fertility such as when approaching the menopause; or, on the other hand, when you want to have a child.

While learning the method should I keep a record of my mucus for a menstrual cycle or for a calendar month?

It is necessary to chart your mucus for a calendar month only. (If ovulation is delayed for a long time in a cycle, the complete cycle may take several months; charting for this length of time would involve much unnecessary abstinence.) One month is sufficient time for you to assess your state of fertility.

How many days during a menstrual cycle is the average couple fertile?

Three to six days. Scientific studies show that the egg lives for about twelve hours, and sperm can maintain their fertilizing capacity for three to five days if supported by the fertile-type mucus from the cervix. Therefore intercourse on the Peak day or within three to five days beforehand, and before the egg dies after the Peak, may result in a pregnancy.

How many days are available for intercourse in a typical twenty-eight day cycle? Does this vary according to the length of the cycle or the circumstances of reproductive life – for example, during breastfeeding, or when approaching the menopause?

Preliminary results from the World Health Organization trial of the method indicate that about half the days of a twenty-eight day cycle are generally available for intercourse. Days of abstinence include the menstrual period, the time when mucus indicates possible fertility, and a safety margin of days to cover individual fertility situations. With experience of the method, couples find they can increase the number of days available for intercourse.

In short cycles, fewer than half the days may be available for intercourse, whilst in long cycles, such as when you are breastfeeding or approaching the menopause, considerably more days are available.

Groups of days of abstinence alternate with groups of days available for intercourse, so that abstinence is not required for lengthy periods in any cycle. This is a decided advantage over other natural methods, and an important psychological help in enabling couples to keep to the guidelines.

When intercourse is inadvisable, don't give up loving altogether. There are many ways to show your love, and with imagination, these days can be as invigorating and fulfilling as the others.

It is often found helpful to think positively about the times without intercourse: the fertile phase, with its potential for conceiving a baby, is a time set aside by mutual decision. Then during the infertile phase, you can enjoy totally relaxed sexual loving, free from contraceptive drugs or devices.

Many couples find that their sexual relationship is revitalized after a short break from intercourse.

You say that sperm can live for up to five days. What if I don't have five days of fertile mucus to warn me that ovulation is approaching?

Sperm cannot pass through the cervix or maintain their fertilizing capacity without the presence of fertile mucus because the vaginal environment is hostile to them.

So, if you have fertile mucus for only two days, or even half a day of the cycle, sperm vitality will be reduced correspondingly. The important thing to remember is that when you see or feel the stringy, lubricative mucus, you should avoid intercourse then, and for three days afterwards. However many days you see or feel the fertile mucus, you will always have sufficient warning of the approach of ovulation by a change from your infertile pattern.

Why is it important to make love only at night in the first part of the cycle before the fertile mucus becomes apparent?

You need to be on your feet for a few hours so that the fertile mucus can make itself felt or seen. Intercourse upon waking in the morning would not enable you to be aware of a night-time change to fertile mucus and so a pregnancy might result. Once ovulation has occurred and a gap of three days set aside, day or night is available for intercourse.

Why do you advise abstinence as soon as the change from infertile mucus to the fertile-type mucus becomes apparent?

It is impossible to predict in any cycle just when ovulation will occur. In a short cycle of say twenty-one days, this may happen on about day seven.

The fertile mucus enables sperm movement to the tubes and maintains sperm vitality for up to five days. Without the mucus sperm fertilizing capacity diminishes rapidly. The rule to avoid intercourse when fertile signs become apparent ensures that sperm cells will not retain their fertilizing capacity until ovulation.

Fertile signs may begin more than five days before the Peak (the average is six days beforehand). Since it will not be known in any cycle how soon ovulation will occur, the rule to defer intercourse from the first point of change may add a day or two of abstinence which, in retrospect, can be seen to have been unnecessary.

In some cycles, mucus may not appear until very close to ovulation. The same rules will apply, because *sperm transport is blocked and vitality declines quickly without the fertile-type mucus*. The only difference is that during such cycles with a small number of fertile days the time of abstinence will be shorter.

You suggest three days of abstinence after the Peak or last day of fertile mucus. But doesn't the egg die within twelve hours of its release? Thus isn't it impossible to conceive so long after ovulation?

Studies show that the Peak, as identified by a woman herself, correlates closely with ovulation. In about 85 per cent of women it occurs within a day of ovulation and in about 95 per cent within two days (see p. 179).

After the Peak, your fertility declines rapidly as the fertile-type mucus is replaced by infertile mucus. A gap of three days after the Peak allows sufficient time for your fertility to decline to zero: within this three days, the egg dies. The three-day gap (Peak rule) is a little excessive in terms of the scientific data on egg and sperm survival times. However it is designed to allow for a margin of error in assessing your Peak.

How much need my partner know about the method?
Should I tell him when I notice the fertile-type mucus so that
he knows we cannot make love?

This is one advantage of a chart. Together you can watch your
mucus pattern emerge. When your partner understands what
it means, he will know when the best times for intercourse are.

Both partners may feel at times that they would like to throw
caution to the wind, even though the mucus indicates fertility.

If a couple has decided in advance that this is not the right
time for a child, they can support and encourage each other to
follow the guidelines. Successful users of the Ovulation
Method have devised many different and individual ways to
indicate that it is the fertile phase – a rose in a vase, a chart in an
accessible place, or a word about the presence of fertile-type
mucus. Many partners experienced in using the method 'just
know'.

This shared approach is extremely important. Couples will
cope with abstinence, but not with confusion.

Can the guidelines be used more flexibly once a woman has
long experience of assessing her own pattern of fertility?

Many women find after using the method for some time that
they can enjoy more freedom for intercourse than the
guidelines recommend and still avoid pregnancy.

The guidelines have been laid down for maximum security
and contain a built-in safety margin. However, couples who
adopt a more flexible approach should be prepared for the
possibility of a pregnancy.

Can I learn the method with confidence from this book?
How important is it to check my mucus observations with a
teacher?

Many women will be able to learn the method from this book.
However some may find it helpful to consult a trained Ovulation Method teacher, especially if their pattern is difficult to

interpret as may be the case after coming off the Pill or when approaching the menopause.

With whom can I check my chart so that I know I am interpreting my mucus signals correctly?

The best person to advise you about your chart is a trained teacher of the Billings Ovulation Method. A full list of accredited teachers is available from the Ovulation Method Centre, 27 Alexandra Parade, North Fitzroy, Melbourne, Australia. (See p. 200 for a list of national centres.) If a teacher is not available in your area, a woman who has successfully used the method should be able to give much good advice.

Doesn't this method take the spontaneity out of love-making?

The use of any natural method means that you can't always have intercourse when you feel like it. To avoid a pregnancy you can't have intercourse when you are fertile. This approach needs to be discussed and mutually agreed upon by partners when they decide to use the method.

Weighed against this are the many days when love-making can be completely spontaneous, free from drugs and devices, and from any doubts about your state of fertility.

What relationship has the fertile-type mucus to ovulation?

From an average of six days before ovulation, mucus begins which soon takes on lubricative, stringy qualities and looks like raw egg-white.

This mucus – the fertile-type mucus – is caused by rising levels of the hormone, oestrogen, acting on the cervix. All the evidence suggests that it is essential for movement of sperm and maintenance of their fertilizing capacity, and is a reliable warning signal that you are fertile.

The Peak of fertility – which corresponds closely with ovulation – is the last day of any sensation or appearance of the fertile-type mucus. *It is not the day of maximum mucus. This is a common error.* (The sensation of lubrication may continue for a day or two after visible mucus disappears – but the continuation of the sensation indicates that you are still fertile.)

How do you account for the changes in the cervical mucus?

A number of studies have investigated the changing nature of the mucus and have linked these changes with hormones. Basically, the different types of mucus are produced in response to different levels of the hormones oestrogen and progesterone. These hormones come from the ovary. They act directly on the cervix to stimulate the formation of the different types of mucus which you will see and feel. The fertile mucus becomes apparent as the egg begins to mature in response to a rising oestrogen level. Following ovulation, progesterone causes the cervix to produce the sticky dense mucus, and a dramatic change in sensation. Photographs on p. 120 show the different characteristics of the mucus.

I can recognize changes in the appearance of my mucus, but I am not confident of my ability to detect changes in sensation. Does this mean I should not use this method?

No. Whilst both the sensation and appearance of the mucus are important indicators of your state of fertility, awareness and recognition of these may take time to develop. Persevere with the method, and take the time to chart your mucus pattern. Many women find that their ability to detect sensations develops rapidly and becomes second nature to them. Studies show that most women can produce a recognizable mucus pattern after only one month of learning the method.

Is the fertile-type mucus always clear?

No, this mucus may be cloudy, or it may be tinged red, pink, or brown, from blood, a few drops of which may be produced at the time of ovulation.

Although the appearance of this mucus varies, its consistency resembles raw egg-white, and it always has the characteristic of slipperiness or lubricativeness. Occasionally, some women see no mucus but feel the lubricating sensation, *indicating that they are fertile*.

Is it always easy to see the mucus?

Most women see, as well as feel, the different types of mucus during their cycles. A very few women say they see very little, if any, mucus but are aware of an unmistakable sensation for which even small amounts of mucus are responsible.

Is it possible to conceive without producing the fertile-type mucus?

All the evidence suggests that fertile-type mucus must be produced by the cervix for conception to occur (see chapter 15). This is because the mucus assists sperm transport and provides the environment in the vagina that is necessary for the maintenance of sperm fertilizing capacity. On the basis of this evidence considerable doubt must be expressed about the possibility of a pregnancy when mucus is not produced.

The importance of fertile-type mucus is now recognized by infertility workers throughout the world. Couples having difficulty conceiving are advised to be alert for mucus with fertile characteristics, and use these days for intercourse.

Does stress affect the mucus pattern?

Stress – perhaps caused by excitement, illness, or an emotional upset – may delay ovulation or cause its complete elimination from your cycle. Travel may also delay ovulation. There is no evidence to indicate that stress speeds up ovulation.

Any delay in ovulation will be mirrored by your mucus. For example, if severe stress occurs in the few days preceding ovulation, you will notice that your fertile-type mucus suddenly stops and is replaced either by an infertile mucus pattern or by dryness.

Because it may be difficult to be sure at such a time whether ovulation has occurred, a gap of three days should be allowed before resuming intercourse, and the Early Day Rules (p. 42) followed until the Peak is recognized. Occasionally severe stress may result in a confused pattern of mucus and it is advisable to postpone intercourse during this time.

Can intercourse trigger ovulation?

Hormonal studies on humans have not been able to establish a relationship between intercourse and ovulation.

If couples don't wish to conceive, intercourse should be deferred as soon as signs of fertility become apparent, and for three days past the Peak.

Can knowledge of my mucus pattern help me identify infection or disease?

Yes, women who get to know their normal body processes are often aware immediately anything goes wrong.

If the mucus pattern changes significantly – for example, there may be a sudden increase in the amount of mucus, or the colour or odour of the mucus may alter – it is a good idea to consult a doctor. An altered pattern may be due to disorders such as polycystic ovaries or infection.

Gynaecologists are paying increasing attention to these changes, for they may indicate an abnormality or disease of the reproductive organs, a hormonal upset or a side-effect of medication. The earlier a disorder is diagnosed, the greater the probability of a successful treatment.

Do any drugs affect the mucus?

Yes, the following drugs alter the mucus pattern, with variable effects in different women:

• Some tranquillizers, e.g. Largactil, by causing raised prolactin resulting in delayed ovulation. (However, when ovulation does occur, it will be recognized by the familiar mucus pattern.)
• Hormones, for example, progesterone and oestrogens.
• Anti-histamines (some women only are affected; individual charting will soon determine this).
• Cytotoxic drugs used in cancer. These prevent mucus production by a direct action on the ovaries.
• Antibiotics. Women taking antibiotics for a severe illness sometimes notice a change in the mucus pattern. This may be an effect induced by the stress of the illness and not the drug. Women on continuous antibiotics for chronic illness can interpret their mucus pattern successfully.

Do vaginal sprays and douches alter the mucus pattern?

Yes. They produce an artificial wetness which may confuse your interpretations of the mucus. They may also cause an allergic reaction or inflammation, resulting in an infective discharge which alters the mucus pattern.

While cleanliness is essential to good health and an important consideration in a sexual relationship, it is unnecessary and inadvisable to use these preparations to clean the vagina. The vagina is self-cleansing, and external washing is quite adequate.

What changes to the mucus can I expect after a curettage? Can I still use the Billings Method effectively?

The stress of a curettage may delay ovulation and therefore postpone the production of the fertile-type mucus.

It is advisable to avoid intercourse until the Peak is recognized because the mucus pattern may be temporarily disturbed and unfamiliar. Then apply the method guidelines as usual.

Women who have recently had a curettage may not feel well enough to enjoy intercourse. If this disinclination is discussed with your partner ahead of time, it can be accepted with understanding.

Is there any reason why my partner and I should not use withdrawal during my fertile time?

Withdrawal is not a good idea for two reasons.

Firstly, your partner may lose a drop of semen before orgasm, and this usually contains sperm, which could lead to an unintended pregnancy.

Secondly, withdrawal is often unsatisfactory for both man and woman. Your partner can't relax because he knows that he has to withdraw before ejaculating; and you can't relax because you know he may fail to do so. The anxiety is pointless because it is now established that fertile mucus outside the vagina enables sperm cells to find their way to the Fallopian tubes and the awaiting egg cell. Penetration is not necessary for conception.

Also, withdrawal usually occurs before a woman reaches, or completes, an orgasm. This can lead to considerable mutual frustration and discontent.

Clinical reports indicate that withdrawal may be responsible for sexual passivity in women who would rather suppress their responses than endure frequently repeated frustration when intercourse stops short of orgasm.

Can I combine physical methods of contraception, such as the condom and diaphragm, with the Ovulation Method?

No. There is a good biological reason for not using barrier methods during your fertile phase. The seminal fluid and vaginal secretions associated with intercourse will tend to confuse your mucus pattern and will make it much more difficult to assess your state of fertility correctly. There is no surer way to avoid a pregnancy than avoidance of intercourse when you are fertile. In addition, all the barrier contraceptives have a method failure rate and using a condom or a diaphragm at the fertile time may result in a pregnancy.

I seem to have only a trace of mucus. Is the amount of mucus produced important?

For conception to occur, it is essential that some mucus is produced, because without it, sperm cannot survive to reach and fertilize the egg. However, often women think they have little or no mucus until they start to keep a daily record. They then become alert to the mucus, and realize that they are producing much more than they had thought.

If, after charting, you find that you are producing only a little mucus, this may be quite normal. Your Basic Infertile Pattern may be one of dryness, and when your level of fertility changes, you will notice a small amount of fertile-type mucus. The sensation will change.

If you are completely dry throughout the cycle, your fertility may be impaired, and it is wise to consult a doctor.

I feel a lot of wetness before making love when I've been dry all day. Is this fertile mucus?

It may be fertile mucus that has just begun to be produced by the cervix. But it may be the lubricating mucus produced by the vagina in response to sexual excitement.

If you check your mucus during the day and in the evening, before you are even thinking about making love, you will gain a clear indication of your state of fertility.

The fertile days are usually heralded by a sticky, cloudy mucus after dry days. Or you may notice a plug of mucus. This pattern changes to a stretchy, lubricative mucus nearer to the Peak. Charting will reveal your individual pattern. You will soon be able to recognize the effect of sexual intercourse on your mucus pattern. A chart which shows the effect of intercourse on the mucus pattern is illustrated on p. 115.

I feel more sexually interested when my mucus is of the fertile-type. Is there a biological explanation for this?

Yes. The mucus is exceptionally lubricative at the time of ovulation, and is therefore ideal for intercourse. This may be the reason for your heightened libido at this time. Other factors which some couples notice are an arousing odour associated with the fertile-type mucus, and a fullness of the tissues around the vagina. These characteristics are due to a high level of oestrogen hormone produced by the ovaries when you are fertile.

After the fertile phase, I sometimes feel uninterested in sexual intercourse. Why is this? Can it be overcome?

The basic reason for this disinclination is hormonal. After ovulation the level of oestrogen hormone declines. This is associated with a decline in the lubricative mucus produced by the cervix, which assists intercourse. Its place is taken by a drier thicker mucus produced by the cervix under the influence of progesterone. The resulting dryness can be overcome by an unhurried preparation for love-making which allows secretions to develop in the glands around the vaginal opening and also allows the vagina to become lubricated.

The level of progesterone hormone increases after ovulation. This is associated with an emotional let-down. 'I couldn't when I wanted to, so now I don't want to' is a frequent initial reaction. You may find that you need to make a conscious effort to be affectionate. This ability is something that grows and a man needs to understand this and encourage its development by special attention at this time.

Hormonal changes during the cycle are only one factor in a woman's feeling of emotional well-being and enjoyment of intercourse. The love-making in the infertile part of the cycle can be very satisfying because it is based on loving consideration by both partners.

Will I become pregnant if I make love on the first day after noticing a change from my Basic Infertile Pattern?

The change from an infertile pattern indicates an alteration in hormone levels and therefore possible fertility. You thus

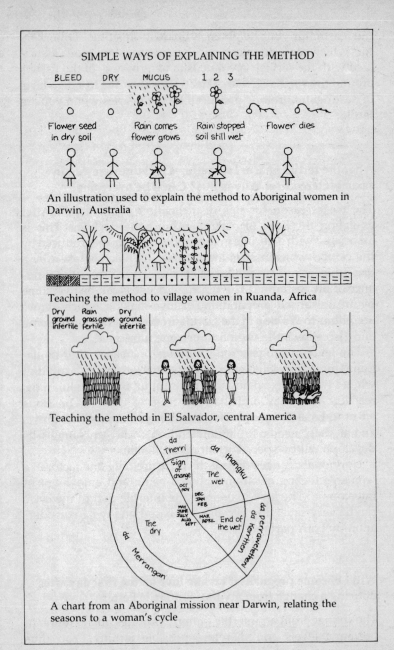

SIMPLE WAYS OF EXPLAINING THE METHOD

BLEED	DRY	MUCUS	1 2 3	
Flower seed in dry soil	Rain comes flower grows	Rain stopped soil still wet	Flower dies	

An illustration used to explain the method to Aboriginal women in Darwin, Australia

Teaching the method to village women in Ruanda, Africa

Dry ground infertile   Rain grass grows fertile   Dry ground infertile

Teaching the method in El Salvador, central America

da Therri
da thangku
Sign of change
OCT NOV
The wet
DEC JAN FEB
MAY JUNE JULY AUG SEPT
MAR APRIL
End of the wet
The dry
da perawchetham
da korrthorn
da Merrangan

A chart from an Aboriginal mission near Darwin, relating the seasons to a woman's cycle increase your chances of becoming pregnant if you have intercourse.

Some couples experiment with these early days of fertile mucus, and find that they do not conceive.

But if couples are strongly motivated to avoid a pregnancy, they should avoid intercourse on any day when the mucus indicates possible fertility, because sooner or later deviation from the guidelines may result in conception. This may come as a surprise to couples who have consistently found such a day infertile.

A friend of mine says she conceived after making love during her period. Is this possible?

It is possible to conceive during your period, particularly if your cycles are very short. The shorter your cycle, the earlier you ovulate, because you ovulate about two weeks before your following menstrual period. For example, if you make love on the sixth day of bleeding and ovulate on day nine of a twenty-four day cycle, you could become pregnant.

Your mucus will warn you of your increasing fertility by becoming stringy and lubricative. However, since it may be obscured by your menstrual bleeding, it is advisable to avoid intercourse while you are menstruating.

It is also worth remembering that the spots of blood that may immediately precede ovulation later in the cycle are sometimes confused with another menstruation. Intercourse at such a time is highly likely to result in conception.

Most books say menstruation happens fourteen days after ovulation, yet you quote a range of ten to sixteen days. Don't most women experience a fourteen day post-ovulatory phase?

About half of all fertile women have thirteen or fourteen day post-ovulatory phases most of the time. The other half tend to have ten to twelve, or fifteen to sixteen, days between ovulation and menstruation. An individual woman tends to keep the same interval of time between ovulation and menstruation.

I have been using the Pill for the past three years. Can I switch to this method immediately?

Yes. The first step is to stop taking the Pill. Then, start to chart your mucus pattern. After about a month's charting you should be able to recognize if you are fertile or infertile. During this month it is advisable to avoid intercourse, so that your pattern is not obscured by seminal fluid or vaginal secretions associated with intercourse. After this time you will be able to use the method guidelines.

Many women are infertile for some months after coming off the Pill, and the mucus pattern will have infertile characteristics which you will soon come to recognize. Any change from this pattern suggests altered fertility, and the need for a brief period without intercourse as your fertility returns. The special circumstances of coming off the Pill are discussed in chapter 9. A chart of a woman who discontinued the Pill is shown on p. 116.

When coming off the Pill, should I wait for my first period before beginning to chart my mucus pattern?

No, it is not necessary to wait for your first period – this may not occur for several months. As soon as you stop taking the Pill, start charting. You will be able to recognize whether you are fertile or infertile from your mucus.

I am twenty-three and my cycles are long and irregular. Do I need hormone treatment to reduce them to the average length in order to use the Ovulation Method?

Irregularity of cycles is no obstacle to using the method. This is because you assess your mucus signals of fertility and infertility on a cycle-by-cycle basis rather than relying on a rigid calendar rule.

There is no need to alter the length of your cycles. Hormone treatment for this purpose is now discouraged by leading medical authorities because it disrupts normal physical and emotional patterns. In some cases, the disturbance caused by hormone treatment may be so great as to result in prolonged infertility. Since these hormone preparations eliminate the normal mucus pattern, it is impossible to use the Ovulation Method while undergoing such treatment.

A possible cause of very irregular cycles is that you are not ovulating. This may be due to a number of factors (see p. 130). If charting your mucus indicates that you are not ovulating, further medical investigation is necessary.

Is it necessary to continue abstinence during menstrual bleeding if your body, over a long period, does not have short cycles?

There is no guarantee that your body will always follow the same pattern. Often the onset of the pre-menopause is marked by a very short cycle in which ovulation occurs during the menstrual bleeding. So, if you do relax the guidelines by having intercourse during menstruation, you leave yourself open to the possibility of a pregnancy.

My cycles average only twenty-one days. Then, very soon after the days of menstrual bleeding, I notice fertile-type mucus. Can I use the Ovulation Method?

Yes, the length of cycle does not alter the applicability of the method.

Your early ovulation, as indicated by the fertile-type mucus, means that you will have few, if any, early infertile days. But intercourse can be resumed from three days after your Peak of fertility and, of course, if cycles are short, your post-ovulatory infertility which is free of all restrictions, returns more frequently.

I have been trying to have a baby for more than a year, but without success. Can I use the Ovulation Method to become pregnant?

To increase your chances of having a baby to the maximum, you will need to follow the method guidelines – in reverse. Once you have read this book carefully and understand the principles of fertility, start to chart your mucus to find out if and when you are ovulating. The fertile-type mucus will indicate your fertile phase. It may not occur in every cycle. The fertile mucus may last for several days or only half a day in a cycle, so you may need to watch carefully for it. Aim to have intercourse every few days whilst keeping a close check on your mucus, and when the fertile mucus becomes apparent, use these days. When the mucus is stringy like raw egg-white, and lubricative, the sperm cells will have the best chance of fertilizing the egg.

Fertility clinics the world over now recognize the importance of the cervical mucus. For example, doctors involved in artificial insemination realize that it is useless to inseminate a woman except when she is producing fertile-type mucus.

Can the Ovulation Method be used to influence the sex of a baby?

The scientific evidence on this is controversial.

Some users say that intercourse early in the development of fertile-type mucus – with no other coitus during that cycle – tends to result in a girl; while intercourse confined to the day of Peak fertility tends to result in a boy.

A recent study in Nigeria appears to confirm this tendency. This study was based on the theory that a single act of intercourse at the Peak would result in a boy; whilst intercourse around the time of the mucus change before the Peak, with no further intercourse until after the fertile phase was over, would result in a girl.

According to the study co-ordinator, Dr (Sr) Leonie McSweeney:[1]

Success in pre-selection of a boy was achieved by 310 couples. Failure in pre-selection of a boy occurred in four couples. Success in pre-selection of a girl was achieved in 90 couples. Failure in pre-selection of a girl occurred in two couples.

Others who have tried to use the method to pre-select the sex of a child have generally achieved a lower success rate. Pre-selection of the sex of a baby is never likely to be 100 per cent reliable.

Will hormone or other treatments enable a woman to produce the fertile mucus and thus help her to conceive?

Use of the chemical, Ethynyl oestradiol, has succeeded in producing mucus with lubricative, stringy qualities. However, success in achieving pregnancies has not followed. Research on this form of treatment is continuing.

What is the reason for a statistically low pregnancy rate in rape?

Statistically, the chances of rape coinciding with ovulation or the fertile-type mucus are slight. It may also be that the severe stress of such an attack would delay the ovulation process; so that the sperm cells die before the egg leaves the ovary. It is often thought that curettage removes the sperm cells. This is not so. The curettage removes the uterine lining, so that if a fertilized egg does eventuate, there is nowhere for it to implant.

It is important for every woman to know the fertile signs, so that in the event of rape she can assess the possibility of conception at once.

Sometimes I see a small blood loss about two weeks before my period. What does this mean?

Such 'spotting' may indicate ovulation. It is due to a high level of the hormone oestrogen acting on the endometrium or lining of the uterus, and causing a seepage of blood through it, a day or two before ovulation.

The blood loss is usually slight and gives the mucus a tinge of colour. Occasionally it is quite heavy, particularly during a long cycle, and it may obscure the mucus. Hence the importance of the guideline to defer intercourse on any day of bleeding, and for three days afterwards. Although the blood loss usually occurs close to ovulation, it is not experienced by a great percentage of women, and is therefore not a reliable guide to ovulation.

I have a chronic discharge due to cysts of the cervix. Can I use the Ovulation Method?

Yes, by charting your mucus daily, you will soon learn to recognize the pattern of mucus associated with a chronic condition. Even when a chronic discharge exists, a change will be noticed in the pattern when the state of fertility alters.

The discharge accompanying cervical cysts is variable and may be a continuous, wet, slippery mucus. The abnormality should be rectified, resulting in the return of your normal pattern.

In the case of an acute infection, such as that caused by the fungus *Candida albicans* (monilia), also known as 'thrush', your mucus pattern will be altered, as it may be by T-mycoplasma, gonorrhoea or trichomonas. These require treatment, during which it is advisable not to have intercourse. This is because intercourse may break up the colonies of organisms and cause them to spread, for example to the urinary system, or to your partner. Local agents used for treating thrush tend to cause drying out of the discharge and the mucus. Therefore wait until after treatment and the return of your normal mucus pattern before resuming intercourse.

Is it possible to ovulate twice in a cycle? Does this affect the reliability of the guidelines?

It is possible to release two or more eggs in a cycle but studies show this always occurs *on the same day*. So all aspects of the Ovulation Method still apply: the guidelines are not affected by multiple ovulation.

During my cycle I sometimes experience pain in the lower abdomen or back, which can be quite sharp. Is this a sign of ovulation?

Some women commonly experience such a pain during their cycles. Studies show that this may be related to the overall rise in hormones associated with ovulation. The pain may be sharp, or dull, rather like a period pain.

The mechanism of this pain production is not fully understood. In many cases it occurs when the oestrogens rise even when ovulation does not occur. It may be due to contractions of muscle tissue in the uterus in response to hormones; or the pain may be due to muscle-sensitizing chemicals (prostaglandins) found in seminal fluid which set off a hormonal response, said to affect the activity of muscles in the female reproductive organs.

Since the pain does not always coincide with ovulation, it is not a reliable guide to fertility.

How accurate is a temperature rise in indicating ovulation? Does keeping a temperature chart help in the recognition of the fertile phase? Is there a place for temperature measurements in natural birth control?

Temperature is not a completely reliable or accurate indicator of ovulation. Studies show that a rise in temperature may occur up to four days before, to six days after, ovulation,[2] although in some cycles it occurs on the day of ovulation. A false high temperature may be caused by a fever. If you rely on this reading for proof of ovulation, you could become pregnant. And in some fertile cycles, no temperature rise occurs around the time of ovulation.

Temperature readings have no value in *predicting* when you will ovulate – a necessity in any effective natural fertility control method.

Another disadvantage is that if you defer intercourse until you see a temperature rise, and if this does not occur until late in your cycle, the time available for intercourse is greatly and unnecessarily restricted.

In addition, there is the disadvantage of the actual taking of temperatures: you are advised to take your temperature for some minutes every morning after at least three hours sleep, and before getting out of bed, eating, or drinking. This can become tiresome and a source of irritation, and in the case of a mother who is disturbed at night by waking children, it may be impossible.

Even when temperature readings are combined with mucus awareness, the result is not always satisfactory. For a temperature rise may not occur until several days after you see or feel fertile mucus. Thus temperature recordings may cause confusion, and can divert attention from the mucus, which is the more accurate guide to your state of fertility.

Under normal circumstances the routine taking of temperature is unwarranted.

However, temperature measurements may prove of value when no recognizable mucus pattern is apparent (for example, due to a defective cervix), or when the mucus is temporarily obscured by an erratic discharge, provided ovulation is occurring.

Where a woman is trying to conceive and is recording a poor mucus pattern, a rise in her basal body temperature will indicate that she is ovulating and that further investigation is necessary.

Might I ovulate but not produce any fertile-type mucus?

Yes, this is possible. The cycle will then be infertile, because the sperm fertilizing capacity diminishes rapidly without the fertile mucus. Clinical investigations show that this situation occurs in some women who have difficulty conceiving. The problem is the subject of intensive research.

It is not uncommon for young women to experience an occasional ovulatory cycle without mucus. And the occurrence of such infertile cycles becomes common in women nearing the menopause, when the cervix becomes unresponsive to rising hormones; this, in part, accounts for declining fertility.

I find intercourse painful and uncomfortable and have been using lubricants to help overcome this problem. Since I wish to have a baby, is this advisable?

The problem of a dry vagina can be overcome by unhurried and loving preparation for intercourse which allows the vagina to produce its own lubricating secretions.

Artificial lubricants often contain chemicals that kill sperm or make the environment of the vagina hostile to them. So it is best to avoid their use if you want a baby.

Lubricants will also tend to obscure the fertile mucus by their artificial wetness, so making it difficult to time intercourse to coincide with your Peak of fertility. If you are anxious to conceive it is important to know that you are most fertile when your mucus is stringy and lubricative, like raw egg-white.

I have had three children in close succession and have not experienced a period during this time. Can the Ovulation Method help me know when my fertility returns after the birth of a child?

Yes; the awareness of your mucus will enable you to recognize when your fertility returns after childbirth. And by following the Ovulation Method guidelines you and your partner will be able to space your children as you wish.

The births of your three children close together indicate that you conceived each time during your first fertile cycle after childbirth.

I am breastfeeding and have no periods yet; so I am relying on my mucus changes to warn me of my first ovulation. However, I seem to be producing wet mucus all the time. Does this mean I am fertile now?

If your mucus is continually wet, and has remained the same day after day for two weeks or more, this is your Basic Infertile Pattern and indicates infertility.

As soon as there is any *change* from this constant situation you will know that your hormone levels are rising. Oestrogens fluctuate for a month or two before your first ovulation and period. The return of fertility depends to a large extent on the age and sucking habits of your baby.

If you wish to avoid a pregnancy, apply the Early Day Rules. If your mucus pattern changes frequently causing confusion, postpone intercourse until the fourth day after you have recognized the Peak. A trained Ovulation Method teacher is the best person to guide you through this time of hormone adjustment.

When preparing for a successful and enjoyable breastfeeding experience with your baby, it is most important that you understand the associated infertility of this period: that it is a time during which you and your partner are free to have intercourse with security. If a temporary period without intercourse is necessary as your fertility returns, frustration can be avoided by couples discussing this possibility ahead of time.

I noticed that when my menstrual periods began after the birth of my daughter, they started about one week after ovulation, as indicated by the fertile-type mucus and the Peak. Would this be a fertile cycle?

The cycle is not a fertile one if menstruation starts less than ten days after ovulation.

This situation is common during and after breastfeeding and is due to the effects of the 'milk hormone' prolactin. A shortened interval between ovulation and menstruation can also occur as you approach the menopause.

My periods come only every few months now as I am forty-three. What should I do about avoiding pregnancy?

If you don't have a period very often, then you are not ovulating very often either, if at all.

You can rely on the mucus from the cervix to inform you of possible fertility. By being alert to mucus changes and by following the guidelines, you can avoid a pregnancy.

After reading this book, chart your mucus for a month,

whilst avoiding intercourse to ensure a clear picture of your mucus pattern. Typically, the pattern is one of long phases of infertility interspersed by occasional episodes of possible fertility.

The recognition of infertility is of paramount importance.

A trained Ovulation Method teacher will help guide you through this phase of your reproductive life if you are having difficulties. She will be able to provide the information to overcome any problems; solutions are usually not difficult.

I am forty-six and my cycles are very irregular. I am worried about becoming pregnant, but my doctor advises against the Pill because I suffer from high blood pressure. Would I be able to use the Billings Method?

Yes; the Ovulation Method is particularly helpful in situations such as yours. Past the age of forty, fertility diminishes substantially, and cycles become irregular as hormones fluctuate.

By charting your mucus you may find that even though your periods continue, you are ovulating rarely and you are infertile most of the time.

So you need to be able to *recognize infertility*. This positive recognition of infertility is a feature of the Ovulation Method not shared by other natural methods such as the Rhythm and Temperature methods.

After charting for a month or so, you will be able to recognize when you are infertile. Any change in the mucus suggests possible fertility. There is no need to be concerned about whether you have reached the menopause. All you need to recognize are the changes in your infertile pattern. Occasionally days of mucus will remind you that your fertility is still fluctuating.

Trials of the Ovulation Method indicate a 'method effectiveness' of between 97 and 99 per cent. What does this mean?

These figures are based on a number of trials throughout the world (see chapter 16). They indicate that if 100 couples use the method *according to the guidelines* for a year, between one and three pregnancies will occur. We don't know why this is so. Sometimes information is withheld until later.

This method effectiveness compares extremely well with other methods: the Pill (99 per cent), Mini Pill (96 per cent), IUD (94 to 99 per cent), Rhythm (53 to 86 per cent).

The actual pregnancy rate in some Ovulation Method trials is about 20 per cent. Why is this?

The vast majority of pregnancies occur when couples knowingly ignore the guidelines. This is often because they are uncertain about the desirability of having children. Other reasons exist which are very complex and personal. Couples are free to use the method as they wish.

A minority of pregnancies result from inadequate teaching, and others when couples misinterpret the mucus. Pregnancies are extremely rare among couples who co-operate with each other, are well informed about the method, and motivated to make it work.

The term 'continuation rate' is often mentioned when fertility control methods are discussed. What is this?

Statistically it refers to the percentage of women still using a method after a given time. The continuation rate for the Ovulation Method has been 98 per cent after four years in a Melbourne study of pre-menopausal women,[3] 80 per cent after one year in India,[4] 99 per cent after one year in another Indian study,[5] and in a US trial 70 per cent after two years.[6]

Are there any devices available to check whether ovulation is imminent or has occurred?

Professor J. B. Brown of Melbourne University is developing a test kit to indicate when ovulation is about to occur, and then to give confirmation.

The hormone levels at which to set the test have been determined with the co-operation of a group of women, most of whom are Ovulation Method teachers. Their phases of infertility and fertility, as assessed by mucus changes, have been correlated with hormonal analyses.

The test will be of particular value in confirming the point of change in the mucus when some abnormality, such as an infection or cervical damage, has altered the normal pattern.

It will also prove helpful to women who are in any doubt about the significance of their mucus, and will therefore provide a reliable teaching aid. It should not be necessary to use it more than once or twice in a cycle.

The test kit will be of great value in providing a quick, easy demonstration of the change from the Basic Infertile Pattern to fertility, and will provide further evidence for the relationship between mucus characteristics and sperm survival.

Other researchers around the world are investigating test tapes or dip-and-read stick systems that measure the levels of various hormones, the viscosity of the mucus, substances in the saliva, or chemicals in the cervical mucus, thus indicating the state of fertility.

Research is also continuing on the development of devices which could predict ovulation by measuring, for example, changes in vaginal blood flow, or the body's electrical charges. These will all need full investigation and careful trial.

For the vast majority of women, their own observation of the mucus is a simple, reliable guide to their fertility: no devices of any kind are necessary.

Learning about fertility in adolescence

When a girl is born, her ovaries each contain half a million or so follicles which are spheres of cells containing all the eggs that will be released during her fertile life.

Only three to five hundred of these will develop into mature eggs. The other follicles degenerate before completing development, many before puberty.

Each girl has her own 'biological clock', centred in the brain, that sets her menstrual cycles in motion. At puberty, generally between the ages of eleven and fourteen in girls, the pituitary gland just below the brain, influenced by the 'clock', signals the ovaries to begin producing the hormone, oestradiol, in sufficient amounts to cause breast enlargement, maturing of the sex organs, and emotional changes. Changes in the uterus also occur which make menstruation possible.

The beginning of the menstrual periods is called the menarche and it usually occurs at about thirteen years of age although it may occur as early as nine or as late as seventeen.

The first year or two is a time of menstrual irregularity for most girls, but then the cycle settles down to a pattern (usually of twenty-three to thirty-five days) from the beginning of bleeding to the last day before the next period begins. This phase of fluctuating hormones plays an important role in growth processes and future reproduction. Natural irregularities of cycle length should on no account be manipulated by the Pill and other hormones to bring about regularity. Women can be quite healthy and have irregular cycles all their reproductive lives; no treatment is necessary.

Most girls do not ovulate for the first year or so after menstruation begins, that is, their ovaries do not release an egg ready for fertilization and a possible pregnancy. The hormones are priming the reproductive system, getting it ready for later fertility.

So in the beginning the signs of fertility may not be present. By knowing about the mucus changes that signal the body's emerging fertility, you can recognize it when it arrives. At first there will be odd episodes of sticky or flaky mucus coming from the vagina. Gradually over several months, the cyclical fertile pattern of slippery, stretchy mucus will be seen. (See chapter 4 where the mucus is described in detail.)

With ovulation the second hormone from the ovary, progesterone, plays its part, producing a change from the fertile mucus pattern.

At times, when ovulation begins, periods may become rather uncomfortable, even sometimes severely painful. Hormone treatment to stop ovulation will stop the discomfort, but such treatment is also known to have dangerous effects reaching into the future, one of the worst being damage to fertility so that your capacity to have a child may be affected. Other treatments are available for pain which are not harmful.

It is important to have a clear understanding of the signs of fertility. This knowledge is healthy and useful throughout life. It is also a good feeling to tune into the rhythms of your body. Moreover it is a matter of some convenience to be able to anticipate the menstrual bleedings. It is also important to know that the fertile mucus is not a disease requiring treatment: it is a normal, healthy sign.

The first four chapters of this book explain the menstrual cycle and describe how you can develop an awareness of when you are fertile by understanding the mucus signs. The mucus – as well as providing the sign – plays a vital role in fertility, because it is essential for maintaining the vitality of the sperm cells. Because the fertile mucus is so favourable to sperm cells, they can travel through it into the body, reach the egg, and fertilize it, even if close sexual contact without actual intercourse has occurred. All this can happen when mucus is present on the body outside the vagina.

Don't trust your mucus record to memory. It is vital to keep a chart while you are learning about your fertility. The pictures on page 120 show what the mucus might look like, but everyone is different, and your pattern may not look quite like this.

Remember that ovulation occurs about fourteen days (the range is ten to sixteen days) before your menstrual period and will be indicated in advance by the mucus. Some women have been led to believe that ovulation always occurs at the midpoint of the cycle. Although this may be true in a twenty-eight day cycle, it is not so in a short cycle of say eighteen days (when ovulation may occur at about day four, perhaps before your period has finished), or in a long cycle of, for example, thirty-five days (when ovulation will take place on about day twenty-one). Within the same woman, the timing of ovulation can vary significantly from cycle to cycle. Hence it is important that you are able to determine, by observing the mucus, when you ovulate *in each cycle*, rather than depending on ovulation occurring at the same time each month.

The female reproductive system matures slowly over several years. A young woman should weigh up the health risks of early sexual activity. It is now known that the risk of cervical cancer is higher among women who start sexual relationships at an early age, and who have more than one sexual partner.[1]

Future fertility can be jeopardized by contracting venereal disease, especially gonorrhoea, if it is not diagnosed early.[2] By the time symptoms develop, or even severe illness, the fine lining of the Fallopian tubes may already be damaged preventing the transport of sperm and egg, or causing the fertilized egg to lodge in the tube instead of the uterus. Damage to tubes from venereal disease cannot be undone. Many people think that venereal disease is a minor disease and easily cured. The truth is that it is a group of serious diseases and some of them cannot be cured easily because the known drugs are increasingly less effective.

If you are involved in a sexual relationship, the greatest dilemma you face could arise from pregnancy. Every act of intercourse in the fertile phase carries with it the possibility of a pregnancy. So the possibility of conceiving a baby needs to be carefully considered if the prospect of intercourse arises.

Some of the information given to adolescents concentrates on methods of contraception, without mentioning that the best and most foolproof method of avoiding pregnancy is abstinence.

If a pregnancy does occur and an abortion is contemplated, it is worth considering that damage to the cervix in order to abort may cause it to become incapable of carrying a later pregnancy to term. Even after the immediate hazards of an abortion are overcome, support and guidance are often needed to recover from this experience and to consider the future realistically and hopefully.

It is worth thinking about possible consequences of these problems now. It is apparent that many young women realize their responsibility for their own body and what happens to it. They are entitled to hope to find one day a partner with views and ambitions similar to their own, instead of giving in to pressure to conform to other people's ideas of when sexual activity should begin.

You will find in the back of the book a list of addresses where the Ovulation Method is taught. Write for the address of a teaching centre near you. You will find the guidance of a trained Ovulation Method teacher helpful in interpreting your mucus pattern. You will enjoy this experience of getting to know yourself and the treasure of your fertility.

9

Coming off the Pill

Coming off the Pill can stimulate a re-assessment of your relationship. Many couples who are postponing or spacing a family, and who are using the Pill as their fertility control method, find themselves in a position where they no longer discuss contraception. There is a tendency to assume that the woman will continue to take responsibility for birth control and to bear its health burden. What may have been intended initially as a temporary contraceptive measure often becomes an ingrained habit, so that decisions about long-term birth control may be deferred indefinitely.

This situation can breed unhappiness and resentment, particularly among women suffering from Pill-induced ill-health. In such a situation, a woman suffering side-effects from the Pill (p. 145) often responds very positively to learning the Ovulation Method and her partner is very happy to have her in good health and spirits again.

If a man acknowledges that part of the responsibility for fertility control rests with him, he is usually willing to accept the co-operation and days without intercourse necessary for successful use of the method.

The first step

If you have decided to use the Ovulation Method, the first step is to discontinue the Pill. You don't have to wait until you finish your present course of tablets ... the sooner you stop taking the Pill, the sooner you can begin to chart your mucus pattern. It is no use trying to learn the method while still taking the Pill; for the synthetic hormones of the Pill alter the mucus pattern.

You do not need to wait until you menstruate or ovulate or your cycles return to their pre-Pill length. Furthermore, irregularity of cycles before you commenced taking the Pill is not a problem since you learn to assess your fertility on a cycle-by-cycle basis.

Charting

You will need to keep a daily record of your mucus for a month while avoiding intercourse and all genital contact. This will ensure that your mucus pattern is not obscured by seminal fluid or vaginal secretions associated with intercourse. A month is sufficient to obtain the necessary information to apply the method whether your fertility has returned or not, or whether you have a period or not.

It will become apparent from your mucus whether you are fertile or infertile. (See p. 37 where the charting is described.) A chart of a woman who stopped taking the Pill is illustrated in Figure 9, p. 116.

What to expect after stopping the Pill

Within a few days of discontinuing the Pill, you will bleed as you normally do after each cycle of the Pill (withdrawal bleed). This is due to the sudden removal of the Pill's synthetic hormones. The lining of the uterus grows in response to the synthetic hormones and is usually shed when these are discontinued.

The next time you bleed may be about one month later. However, not all women menstruate so soon. Typically studies have found that after the initial withdrawal bleed, 30 per cent of women coming off the Pill menstruate within thirty days, a further 60 per cent menstruate within sixty days, another 8 per cent menstruate within two to six months, and 2 per cent do not menstruate until after six months.[1]

There is no way of predicting how long it will take an individual woman's body to return to normal, and for her natural ovulatory cycles to resume. For most women ovulation usually returns after a few cycles. Some may ovulate the first cycle after stopping the Pill: so it is necessary to be watchful for signs of fertility this first month.

Prolonged delays in ovulating occur most commonly among young women using the Pill, and those prone to irregular periods before starting to take the Pill. Although this anovulatory situation is not a threat to health, it makes conception impossible, and suggests a significant metabolic disturbance. Treatment with fertility drugs is often successful in re-starting ovulation and menstruation, and about 50 per cent of women conceive after treatment.[2] As indicated in chapter 12, it is wise to allow at least twelve months for the natural cycles to resume before contemplating fertility drugs.

The mucus after coming off the Pill

The type of Pill you have been using will affect the mucus pattern that you now see. It is most likely that during the first month of charting you will recognize a mucus pattern that indicates infertility.

This infertile pattern will be one of two types. Either you will see no mucus, and experience dryness, or you will have an unchanging mucus that is sticky and scant, or continuous and wet and that looks milky or watery. Different women have their own ways of describing this infertile mucus; however a characteristic they always notice is its unchanging nature.

Both these situations are described as a Basic Infertile Pattern. The first is a Basic Infertile Pattern of dryness, the second, a Basic Infertile Pattern of mucus. This mucus – or lack of it – that signals *infertility* remains the same day after day, without change.

Some women experience a wet discharge that varies significantly from day to day. In such circumstances it is advisable to have a medical examination as this type of mucus may be caused by a damaged cervix, requiring treatment.

The first ovulation after coming off the Pill

Initially, the body may make several attempts to ovulate, and these are recognizable by a change from the Basic Infertile Pattern. The hormone levels may rise and fall again without reaching the level necessary for ovulation. Each rise is associated with a mucus change.

The change may take the form of an altered mucus sensation or appearance, or the occurrence of spotty bleeding. You will know you have not ovulated because of the failure to menstruate within ten to sixteen days of such changes.

Because any of these changes could lead to ovulation, it is important to observe the guidelines described in the following pages. Often the first ovulation after coming off the Pill is accompanied by abdominal pain, severe in some women. However, pain is an unreliable indicator of ovulation, and should not be allowed to contradict your mucus signals.

As you become more aware of your individual mucus pattern, the infertile mucus – whether flaky, sticky, cloudy, or wet, and the same day after day – can be distinguished from any mucus that is different. Recognition of the initial infertile pattern, and avoidance of intercourse during – and for three days after – a change in the pattern, will enable you to see your fertility return without conceiving.

Most women using the Ovulation Method for the first time after taking the Pill will need a few normal cycles to be able to recognize confidently the Peak of fertility.

Naturally it is helpful when learning the method to talk with other women who successfully use it.

Applying the method

After the initial month's charting and, if possible, with the guidance of an experienced teacher to help you interpret your pattern, you will be in a position to apply the method. The guidelines for avoiding a pregnancy are:

MENSTRUATION   Avoid intercourse and all genital contact

on days of heavy bleeding. (The bleeding may obscure fertile-type mucus which may occur during menstruation in short cycles.) If you do not recognize fertile-type mucus and a Peak prior to menstruation, avoid intercourse for three days following bleeding.

THE BASIC INFERTILE PATTERN   During dry days or days of your characteristic infertile-type mucus, alternate evenings are available for intercourse. If ovulation is delayed, you will experience a lengthy time during which these Early Day Rules are applied. By leaving a gap of a day after intercourse you ensure that your mucus pattern is not obscured by seminal fluid or vaginal secretions associated with intercourse. Use of the night for intercourse, rather than the early morning or day, enables you to form an accurate assessment of your fertility through mucus observations during the day.

THE CHANGE   On any day of mucus that differs from your characteristic infertile pattern, or when spotty bleeding occurs, avoid intercourse then, and for three days afterwards. If no Peak has been identified, continue confining intercourse to alternate evenings.

The Peak of fertility is the last day of fertile characteristics of the mucus, that is of stringy or slippery mucus. The day afterwards, stickiness or dryness will begin.

FERTILE-TYPE MUCUS AND THE PEAK   After you recognize fertile-type mucus and the Peak, allow a gap of three days. Thereafter, until your next menstrual period, intercourse day or night as desired will carry no risk of a pregnancy.

IF YOU ARE USING THE METHOD TO HAVE A CHILD   It is advisable to avoid conception for three or four months after coming off the Pill.[3]

This is because there is a tendency to miscarry for several months after using contraceptive hormones. However, those pregnancies that do not miscarry usually proceed normally.

Your chances of achieving a pregnancy are maximized by timing intercourse to coincide with the fertile mucus Peak.

'I stopped taking the Pill because my husband and I wanted to start a family.

We were warned not to attempt to conceive for some months to avoid the possibility of a miscarriage. During this time we learned and practised the Billings Method.

I didn't see any fertile mucus until two months after coming off the Pill; but when it came I had no trouble picking it. Just like clockwork, I had my first menstrual period thirteen days later.

My fertility was back and I felt like cheering. Not only could I have a child, but I felt excited about my new knowledge of how my body worked.'

The method in the balance

Many women who give up the Pill do so after the age of thirty-five when the risk of side-effects increases. These potential risks to health include thrombosis, heart attacks, and high blood pressure (pp. 147–8).

Couples may then feel themselves plunged into a dilemma about fertility control. Should they change to another artificial method of contraception which may disrupt the body's rhythms; or can a natural method provide the solution?

The prospect of some days of abstinence may require some readjustment for a couple used to the Pill. Times of abstinence necessary to avoid pregnancy are, however, compensated for by days of complete sexual freedom.

The temptation to increase the opportunities for intercourse by using barrier contraceptive methods during the fertile phase instead of making full use of infertile days should be resisted, particularly if there is an important reason to avoid pregnancy. Any genital contact, whether barriers are used or not, will confuse the mucus pattern, and increase the possibility of a pregnancy at the fertile time.

Switching to the Ovulation Method brings with it many benefits to health. During the initial month of charting and in the following months, you will probably notice that any vaginal infections clear up. These are commonly associated with Pill use.

Many women experience a psychological lift and an immediate improvement in their moods. For the Pill may contribute to irritability, depression, headaches, and loss of libido.

It is not uncommon to hear women who have changed to the Ovulation Method after being on the Pill talk of a deep satisfaction at tuning into the rhythm of their cycles for the first time. By understanding your fertility, you build up a store of valuable knowledge of your body that will be of benefit for the whole of your fertile life.

'After six years on the Pill, and having developed blood clots in my legs, I was strongly advised by my doctor to come off the Pill. This left us in a difficult situation. My husband and I long ago had decided that our family of three was as many as we could cope with. The prospect of an unreliable method of contraception was extremely upsetting and stressful for us both. Then we heard about the Billings Method. Until I became confident about recognizing my mucus signals, it was difficult and unsettling. But after a few months when my cycles were back to normal and I was confident in my ability to interpret my mucus, I was far happier and more relaxed than I had been for years.'

10

Breastfeeding and the Billings Method

Breastfeeding and the Ovulation Method complement each other. Mother, father and baby all benefit.

After birth, most women experience a period of natural infertility, prolonged for months or even years if a mother breastfeeds her baby. Nature's plan seems to enable you to care for your baby without the demands of another pregnancy too soon. But once the need for your milk diminishes, your body responds by ovulating.

The Ovulation Method enables you to recognize the months of infertility, so that you can enjoy a sexual relationship free from contraceptive devices or anxiety about the possible effects of the hormones in the Pill on your milk and your baby.

Ovulation is likely to occur before your first menstruation, so it is extremely important to develop as early as possible an awareness of the mucus that signals ovulation.

In the same way, women who are not breastfeeding following a birth, or who have suffered a miscarriage, can use their mucus signals to recognize the shift from infertility to fertility. Fertility usually returns within six weeks of the birth if the baby is not breastfed.

'I found it a great relief to be free from worry about condoms, dia-phragms, IUDs, or the Pill, while my baby and I were getting to know each other, and the family was making the inevitable adjustments following a birth.'

'Looking back on all those months, I wish I had known about the OM. We used everything and I was infertile all the time.'

Breastfeeding and the Pill

For many years, the Pill in various forms, and contraceptive injections, have been given to large numbers of breastfeeding mothers. Little consideration has been given to the possible harmful effects of the artificial hormones from contraceptives which may be transferred to babies in breast milk. However a shift away from this practice is now apparent.

This follows careful studies of breast milk which show that both its quality and quantity tend to be detrimentally affected by contraceptive medications (see p. 150). This disturbance has resulted in babies being weaned at an early age, which increases their risk of infection.

Other drugs may also impair the quality of breast milk. The avoidance of all drugs, if possible, during breastfeeding is a healthy practice.

How long are you likely to be infertile while breastfeeding?

The number of months you will be infertile will depend on several factors, including the extent to which your baby demands your breast milk, and on your physical and psychological make-up.

A study of eighty breastfeeding mothers has shown that those who allow the baby to depend on breast milk entirely for nutrition for six months and partially breastfeed thereafter, and who also use the breast as a pacifier, are not likely to ovulate for twelve months after birth.[1]

In Africa, the continuation of breastfeeding of children up to about the age of five in short bursts during the day and at night, enables births to be spaced naturally at intervals of about four years.[2]

Another study of the mothers of forty-two completely breastfed babies shows that none was fertile (as assessed by hormone analysis) within six months of birth. Two of the mothers menstruated without ovulating during this time.[3]

However, if solids are introduced within the first few

months of life, or if mothers are particularly anxious about their breast milk supply, or if the supply of breast milk diminishes for any reason, ovulation is likely to occur sooner.

The key to successful fertility control is to make no assumptions, leave nothing to chance. Watch your mucus carefully, and observe the Ovulation Method guidelines.

What causes this infertility during the breastfeeding period?

Oestrogens are at a low level while you are breastfeeding. This is due to the effect of the hormone, prolactin, which controls breast milk production.

As time goes by, the pituitary gland at the base of the brain starts to switch off prolactin production. Gradually the hormone cycle leading to ovulation takes over. This may occur in a series of stop/start events, as if the body is trying to ovulate. You can see these hormone fluctuations reflected in changes in your mucus. Do not presume the first bleeding you see is menstruation. Light bleeding or spotting may be due to a rise in oestrogens coinciding with ovulation and a return of fertility.

Breast milk production

Sucking sets in motion a reflex chain of events along nerve pathways involving the brain, the pituitary gland, and the breasts. Then the hormone, oxytocin, is released from the pituitary and causes the 'let-down' reflex. This involves a flow of milk from the nipple as special cells around the milk ducts contract. Even the sight or smell or thought of the baby can initiate this very sensitive reflex.

Prolactin, which is responsible for the continuing production of milk, has already been at work, in conjunction with oestrogen and progesterone, causing the growth of glandular breast tissue in preparation for feeding. This hormone continues to operate in response to the baby's sucking.

The sucking skill of the baby develops at the same time as breast growth during pregnancy.

Pictures of a fourteen-week-old foetus often show the thumb being sucked. In this way tiny cheek and mouth muscles are exercised, and the complicated sucking mechanism practised.

The instant and vigorous sucking of the baby when put to the breast after birth often leads parents to exclaim that their child 'knows what to do'. In fact, the baby has been practising for months. Mothers feeling they ought to stop thumb-sucking should realize they are dealing with a long-standing habit.

After birth, if mothers wish to breastfeed, it is desirable that they have access to their babies for feeding according to need. The practice of sedating mothers for a prolonged period to ensure sleep, together with injudicious additions of breast-milk substitutes in the hospital nursery, has been the cause of many breastfeeding failures. Breasts engorged with milk after a long sleep cannot be emptied by a baby who is not hungry, and soon an over-abundance of milk is converted to an inadequate supply. The milk supply is further threatened if a mother becomes anxious when she is told she has 'not enough milk' by a nurse who is conducting test feeds. 'Why bother?' a friend or relative may ask. And the baby goes home on the bottle.

Breast milk is tailor-made for the baby's needs. For the first few feeds, a substance called colostrum is produced by the breasts. This prepares the baby's digestive tract for later milk, and supplies important antibodies to protect against infection. Breastfeeding helps protect the baby from developing allergies to foreign proteins in these first few weeks when the digestive tract is vulnerable. Colostrum is also of benefit to the delicate skin of the nipples, and should not be washed away with soap and water.

Patterns of mucus during infertility

By careful observation, you can learn to recognize your Basic Infertile Pattern while you are breastfeeding.

It doesn't matter if you have not used the Ovulation Method before – you can learn to recognize your infertile pattern by making daily observations.

If you are infertile, your pattern may be:

• Dry all the time – no mucus at all
• The same type of mucus day after day
• Days of infertile-type mucus interspersed with dry days. In this case the characteristics of the mucus remain the same. After observing for two weeks it can be seen that every time the mucus appears it is the same kind of mucus. While the infertile-type mucus may vary from woman to woman, the key to its recognition is its *unchanging pattern*.

Thus a woman may notice a milky wet discharge every day for months on end. Another woman may record flaky, dry or sticky mucus which becomes very familiar as it is noticed each day. Awareness becomes second nature and changes can be picked up and evaluated in relation to her now familiar Basic Infertile Pattern.

During this prolonged phase of infertility, couples may need new insights about how to achieve satisfying intercourse. One common problem is an excessively dry vagina due to reduced production of mucus by the cervix. This can be overcome by an unhurried and loving preparation for intercourse, which allows the vagina to produce lubricating secretions.

It is valuable to realize that intercourse does not depend solely on a raised level of oestrogen hormone to be emotionally and physically satisfying; loving consideration between partners is extremely important. Sensitive nervous reflexes operate which are dependent upon emotional as well as physical stimulation.

Especially loving preparation for intercourse is helpful during the menopause later in life, when a similar dryness may occur. It can readily be seen how the successful management of the infertility of breastfeeding can be a good preparation for menopause when oestrogens are also low.

Charting the mucus pattern

You should begin to keep a record of your mucus from three weeks after the birth when blood loss (lochia) tends to stop. (See p. 37 where the method of charting is explained.) Even though infertility may continue for a considerable time, charting is recommended because it increases your awareness of the mucus signals so that any change is readily noticed. You become familiar with a pattern that indicates infertility.

While charting, it is helpful to describe your mucus observations and sensations in your own words. Also record the number of feeds each day, the longest interval between feeds, any alteration in the feeding routine or sickness, teething and irritability of the baby. This will help you (and an Ovulation Method teacher, if one is available) to assess accurately the state of your fertility.

Mothers of young babies who are fully breastfed, thriving and contented and where the breast is used as a pacifier or comforter, are unlikely to be fertile. If your baby is dependent entirely on your milk for nutrition, is sucking frequently, and on demand, you will probably not ovulate or menstruate for several months.

Under these circumstances you can safely have intercourse according to inclination, apart from the days excluded by the Early Day Rules (p. 42). These include the day following love-making, when your mucus pattern may be obscured by seminal fluid or vaginal secretions associated with intercourse, as well as any days of bleeding, or days when there is any change in the mucus pattern.

If you are partially breastfeeding, or your baby is three months or older, or your periods have returned, you will need to *defer intercourse for two or three weeks while charting*, in order to gain a clear picture of your mucus pattern, and thus of your state of fertility.

After this, if your pattern indicates that you are still infertile, you can safely have intercourse on alternate nights. It is also advisable to confine intercourse to the evenings so that your assessment of fertility is based on a full day's mucus pattern (for the fertile mucus may begin during the early hours of the morning before it is apparent to you).

Some couples attempt to gain more opportunities for intercourse by using a condom or diaphragm without allowing a clear day following intercourse. However intercourse with these devices will result in secretions which may obscure your mucus pattern.

The chart showing the return to fertility of a woman breast-feeding her baby is illustrated on p. 118.

The return of fertility

Any change in your mucus, or any bleeding, may signal a change in your hormone balance and a return of fertility.

You need to be particularly observant for changes in the mucus pattern when:
• Night feeds are discontinued
• Complementary feeds with infant milk formulas are introduced
• Solids are included in your baby's diet
• Your baby's feeding pattern is altered due to sickness or irritability, such as during teething
• Weaning is taking place, and afterwards.

All these events may trigger hormonal changes which set in train the process of ovulation, and thus the return of fertility.

Menstruation will probably not be the first sign of the return of your fertility. You may ovulate before your first period, so you need to watch your mucus carefully.

The first period is often quite heavy, particularly when it is not preceded by ovulation.

Some cycles after your long phase without periods may be anovulatory, that is, no egg will be released. This tends to be the case if menstruation returns within the first nine months after birth.[4]

Or you may experience cycles with a post-ovulatory phase of less than ten days. These cycles are infertile. The reason for this shortened interval between the mucus Peak and the next menstrual period may be an interaction between a raised level of the hormone, prolactin, which stimulates milk production, and your levels of oestrogen and progesterone hormones. Soon after ovulation returns, your cycles will return to a familiar length.

The first sign of any change in your state of fertility may be intermittent days of mucus interrupting a Basic Infertile Pattern of dryness. You may not ovulate, for your body may be 'practising' for the full return of fertility.

If you are watching your mucus, you will usually be warned of the return of fertility well in advance. A study of forty-two breastfeeding mothers showed that thirty-eight had six or more days of fertile-type mucus before ovulation, which was confirmed by hormone measurements.[5]

If the mucus changes, the safest approach is to avoid intercourse on these days of changed mucus and for three days afterwards. This is also the best policy for any day of spotting or bleeding which will tinge the mucus with blood, giving it a pink or brown appearance.

Some women begin regular menstruation early (within the first six weeks) even while breastfeeding totally. Recognition of the mucus pattern and application of the guidelines will enable you to control your fertility in this situation.

If in doubt about possible fertility, it is wise to wait and watch for a few weeks. This period of abstinence presents little problem if couples are prepared for it, and it is usually readily accepted because of the freedom and security made possible by the Ovulation Method in the preceding months.

When ovulation finally occurs it will be associated with the fertile-type mucus. If the cycle is fertile, menstruation will occur ten to sixteen days after ovulation. By carefully observing your mucus signals, this first menstruation after birth can be predicted accurately; an encouraging sign that you are mastering the method.

Maintaining your milk supply

Sometimes babies themselves seem to be aware of the body's attempts to ovulate. They may become irritable and show less inclination for breast milk close to ovulation, when the taste and smell of the milk alter. Menstruation also seems to be associated with some protest by the baby.

Many mothers notice that they are producing less breast milk than usual when their babies are about three months old. The baby's weight gain is suspended, and signs of returning fertility – such as intermittent days of lubricative mucus – may become evident.

Introducing solids or canned baby foods or extra milk at this stage may prematurely halt your milk production. This is the time for some mothering of mother. It is often very helpful if those who are close to you can enable you to devote all your time and attention to your baby. Twenty-four hours in bed, with frequent breastfeeds, is invaluable if you are to maintain your milk supply.

With frequent breastfeeds, extra fluids, nourishing food and rest, the flow of breast milk improves and again becomes adequate. This postpones the onset of fertility and the infertile pattern returns. Once past this three-month hurdle, breastfeeding usually returns to normal, and infertility is prolonged.

Another episode like this frequently occurs when babies are about nine months old. If you and your baby wish to continue breastfeeding at this stage, increased opportunities for sucking and a few days rest usually provide the key.

Britain's Department of Health and Social Security recently published a report on infant feeding in which it recommended that the introduction of solids should be delayed until four to six months.[6]

As long as you are well-nourished and your baby is gaining weight, is happy, and contented, there is no need to introduce solids until the baby is at least four months.

The 'educational diet'

The need for an 'educational diet' is often made obvious by babies themselves.

At about five months of age, they often show interest in the various tastes and textures of foods that others are eating.

Small amounts of solids introduced into your baby's diet will not greatly alter your mucus pattern, as long as the baby's fluid and main calorific requirements are met by breast milk. These eating experiences, which are social as well as educational, are preparing babies to accept adult food with pleasure later on.

Nutritionally speaking, milk should remain the most important component of a baby's diet for nine months to a year. Some babies resist the introduction of other food and prefer to go on sucking. Babies display individual behaviour, and some seem to require substantial amounts of solid foods for months before others.

Weaning

The return of fertility may be prompted by a reduced number of feeds, as the baby is given or demands additional food and other fluids. It may also closely follow any ill health you or your child experience when either insufficient breast milk, or inadequate demand, leads to a reduction of breast milk production.

The effect of weaning on the mucus pattern differs from woman to woman.

If weaning is gradual, or the baby is encouraged to wean himself or herself, there may be several patches of fertile-type mucus before ovulation occurs. For a short time the pattern may be confusing. The sensible solution is to postpone intercourse temporarily until the pattern is clear.

Once weaning is completed ovulation usually follows quickly; this is recognizable by the presence of the fertile mucus and the Peak. Note particularly the change in sensation. Not every woman will *see* abundant mucus.

'I fed my baby for three months. Then he became very cross and cried a lot. I was using the Ovulation Method and after a few weeks I suddenly had a period. That was the beginning of the end. The baby refused my milk and I put him on some bottle feeds. He seemed so hungry. I then noticed a lot of mucus. The baby kept refusing the breast. The mucus stopped. I knew I was going to have a period – which I did. By this time there was very little breast milk left, so I

finished feeding. My cycles then returned to normal. I was told I could have persevered with more frequent feeds, as babies sometimes act in this way at about three months especially when mucus, or menstruation, returns. Next time I will try to encourage more sucking. I am sorry that I had to stop so soon. It wasn't hard to pick my Peak and to understand what was happening with my fertility even though it was the first time I had really noticed mucus.'

Applying the mucus guidelines

Until now, you will have been using guidelines that apply to an infertile pattern. With the return of ovulation and menstruation it is necessary to learn to recognize the Peak of fertility and to apply the Peak rule.

Charting for a month without intercourse will enable you to interpret your pattern accurately, and will provide information about your fertility which will be of benefit for the rest of your fertile life.

Sometimes when cycles begin, a pattern of mucus discharge which indicated infertility while you were breastfeeding will now be replaced by something quite different. For example, a Basic Infertile Pattern of continuous mucus may now be replaced by a Basic Infertile Pattern of dry days. The important point here is that a type of mucus that indicated infertility while you were breastfeeding does not necessarily indicate the same thing once normal cycles have returned.

This is a new set of circumstances, which is why a month of charting without intercourse is necessary.

After the initial month of charting your mucus pattern, continue daily observations and apply the guidelines:

• Avoid intercourse on days of bleeding.
• Use alternate nights for intercourse if there is no visible mucus and the sensation is dry.
• Avoid intercourse as soon as mucus becomes apparent, and for three days following the return of dryness. This three-day margin allows the pattern to become either obviously fertile, or to indicate infertility.
• When the Peak symptom is recognized, postpone

intercourse for three more days. After this the rest of the cycle is available day or night.

'My first period arrived when my first child – Mary – was sixteen weeks old. By the time she was weaned at nine months, I'd had four cycles; the first lasting forty-three days, then thirty-nine days, thirty-eight days, and thirty-six days. As soon as the weaning was complete, I reverted to my usual cycle of twenty-eight days. Mary had slept through the night from ten weeks, and had started an educational diet at three-and-a-half months.

Having successfully fed Mary, I didn't doubt my ability to do the same with Lucy. However, I underestimated the demands of a two-year-old when trying to breastfeed a new baby.

Lucy had nothing but breast milk until she was six months old. I started weaning her at eight months, and it was then that I got my first period. Forty-three days later I had my second period. From then on my cycles returned to the usual length.

When Lucy was three, Loretta arrived on the scene. I learned the Ovulation Method while breastfeeding her. She turned out to be a child that scarcely ever slept. Her consistent pattern was little feeds often. She reminded me of Pavlov's dogs – every time the telephone rang she regarded it as feed time.

This frequent sucking had the effect of keeping me infertile for seventeen-and-a-half months. I didn't introduce her to solids until she was six months old, and until that time I didn't note any mucus symptoms at all; from then on I occasionally had patches.

It was interesting to note that when Loretta was twelve months old we had a caravan holiday for two weeks. Because she was fidgety in the car whilst travelling, I fed her much more frequently throughout that two weeks and, as a result, I had a fortnight entirely free of mucus.

However, when the holiday was over and we settled back to normal, I started to get patches of mucus from time to time. I was able to predict my first period by recognizing the Peak symptom after two years without menstruating, including the time of my pregnancy.

Around the time my periods returned, Loretta gave up nursing in the day time, but continued to nurse at bedtime for another twelve months or so. Eventually at two-and-a-half years, she and I had a long talk and finally she agreed to wean.'

11

Approaching the menopause

Woman is rare among creatures in that she outlives her reproductive capacity.

From the age of about fifty, most women are infertile, with twenty-five years or so of life remaining. The change from fertility to infertility is usually gradual, occurring over a number of years. This period of change is referred to as the 'change of life' or 'climacteric', and is commonly marked by menstrual cycles that are extremely variable in length, and by mucus episodes that are increasingly less frequent.

The change of life often presents problems for a woman and her husband. Irregularity of cycles as the menopause approaches has caused some couples to abstain from intercourse for months or even years. This creates severe stress on relationships, resulting in feelings of rejection and confusion for both.

Sometimes contraceptive medication is used for the first time. Or sterilization is undertaken, or a hysterectomy accepted on the most slender of gynaecological indications . . . *all at a time when a woman is infertile most of the time and soon to be totally infertile.*

At the menopause, a woman can be overwhelmed by feelings of worthlessness, and she may view the future without enthusiasm. She may become withdrawn and introspective, feeling that nobody cares much about her. Bursts of irritability – unreasonable even in her own estimation – are often brushed aside by relatives with the remark 'she'll get over it'. Family members may be mystified and hurt by the change in her disposition. A partner may find it simpler to go his own way, not realizing that her outbursts are a cry for help, and that a gift of flowers, a new dress, a valentine, or an invitation out to dinner, would be appreciated greatly – especially if he could also encourage her to discuss her problems and anxieties in an atmosphere of loving understanding.

At such a time, a woman may see the need to adjust her role, both in society and the family.

She may not feel very interesting, because people seem less interested in her. She may put on weight and feel lethargic and unattractive. Sexual inclination may decline due to physical causes. Heavy periods may result in anaemia, fatigue and depression. Falling oestrogens may have caused dryness of the vagina tending to make intercourse painful. It is not uncommon now for sexual problems which have been suppressed during the active, reproductive years to come to the surface, the scales having been tipped by these unpleasant physical experiences. There may be feelings of inadequacy with an overlay of guilt. Very often the lines of communication have come adrift and some of the problems are purely imaginary. It may be that her partner is more demanding for intercourse because he feels that he is losing his youth, or because she is refusing him and therefore seems to be unloving. This paradoxical situation of poor satisfaction followed by increased sexual demands results in misunderstanding on both sides.

On the other hand, there may be increased sexual inclination on the woman's part, and the couple must adjust to this.

Loving communication between partners can overcome many difficulties. Other positive steps to overcome problems of the menopause are discussed later in this chapter. Of course, in many instances, couples adjust happily to the new situation.

It is impossible and misleading to generalize. For while the menopausal years may bring some problems, many women find opportunities for a creative and fulfilling lifestyle with major family responsibilities over, worries about an unexpected pregnancy eliminated, and with more time to follow their own interests.

The Ovulation Method in the pre-menopause

The Ovulation Method of fertility control can provide security during this time of changing fertility.

If a woman has not used the Ovulation Method before this need not prove an obstacle.

> It is not necessary to predict the end of fertility: the key to successful fertility regulation at this stage is *positive recognition of the infertility* which will eventually become absolute.

A woman can recognize whether she is fertile or infertile from her cervical mucus. If any difficulties arise, a skilled teacher of the method, or another woman who has successfully used the method, will be able to help her through this time of irregularity.

'At forty-five, with my cycles becoming increasingly long and irregular, my life seemed to be turning into a monstrous game of roulette. Would a chance pregnancy result from an occasional act of lovemaking? I wondered anxiously.

My doctor cheerfully told me that I couldn't conceive even if I tried. But when I consulted another doctor he advised the Pill.

When I heard about the Ovulation Method I did not think I could use it because of the lack of any apparent mucus pattern. I could recall mucus resembling raw egg-white occurring perhaps two years ago, but certainly not in recent times.

By keeping a careful record for the next four weeks and by being alert to my mucus subsequently, I knew that I was infertile. This knowledge has given me a new peace of mind and release from unnecessary abstinence.'

Events leading to the menopause

The decline of fertility usually occurs gradually as the functions of the ovaries and cervix change. Most available eggs have matured and left the ovary and although the lining of the uterus may continue to build up and break away and menstruation may continue for months or years due to fluctuating hormone levels, ovulation is occurring less and less frequently.

Statistically, once you reach middle age you are in an age group of low fertility. Studies show that between the age of forty-five and fifty years, only one woman in 700 is able to become pregnant; and after the age of fifty, the figure drops to about one in 25 000.[1]

Typical patterns of changing fertility

The physiological patterns of the pre-menopause vary from woman to woman. However some experiences are common. These include the following:

• Menstrual periods may stop without warning and not begin again. The menopause is the name given to the end of the menstrual periods.

• Cycles may become extremely irregular and vary in length from as short as seventeen days to six months or more; and the amount of menstrual bleeding may likewise vary considerably.

• Ovulation may occur infrequently, although menstrual periods may continue. Do not rely on menstruation as a guide to your fertility. Periods may continue for months or years beyond your ability to conceive.

• Production of the fertile-type mucus by the cervix may stop, even though you may still be ovulating and menstruating. The absence of fertile-type mucus means that you are infertile since this mucus is essential if the sperm cells are to retain their fertilizing capacity and reach the egg.

• The nutritive lining of the uterus – the endometrium – may be shed within ten days of the Peak. This premature breakdown of the endometrium – resulting in an infertile cycle – is due to a fall in hormones produced by the corpus luteum (p. 24). Several factors may be responsible.

Variations between women

The length of the change of life and the severity of associated conditions vary considerably between women. It may extend over months or years, during which fertility may seem to disappear, only to return again months later.

It is impossible to predict when your fertility will finally end, although your pattern may be similar to that of your mother and sisters. The time of the menopause is not related to when your menstrual periods first began, or to the number of children you have.

Assessing your state of fertility

A full medical history will indicate your state of fertility. Factors to be taken into account include:
• Age. If you are forty-five or older you are statistically much less likely to become pregnant.
• Number of children and miscarriages. This is some indication of overall fertility.
• Age of youngest child. This indicates when you were last proven to be fertile. But it does not necessarily tell you anything about subsequent fertility.
• Previous fertility control methods used. Women who have used the Pill and IUD tend to become infertile earlier.
• Recent lengths of menstrual cycles, compared with those you experienced five or ten years ago.
• Approximate date of the onset of irregularity of the cycles.
• Changes in menstrual bleeding, such as reduced or prolonged blood loss, or the presence of blood clots associated with heavy bleeding. Excessive bleeding may cause anaemia and consequent fatigue. Painful periods may have once been the rule. Now many or all are painless.
• Bleeding between periods. This is more common in long pre-menopausal cycles. It sometimes coincides with ovulation, and may be an unfamiliar experience.
• Changes in breast pain or tenderness. Breast tenderness may become very severe, disturbing sleep and lasting for two or three weeks in any particular cycle; or if previously you have

been accustomed to a feeling of soreness, fullness, and lumpiness in the breasts for a few days before menstruation, this may no longer occur. The disappearance of this breast tension can often be related to a decline in the production of fertile-type mucus.

• A temperature record may indicate, by absence of a rise, that ovulation is not occurring in certain cycles.

• Hot flushes. These are brief events, during which a feeling of heat suddenly rises up the body to the head, producing redness of the neck and face and generalized perspiration, which quickly subside. The flushes may occur as many as thirty times a day, and then disappear for several weeks. Or they may not occur at all. They may happen during the day or night, in severe cases causing drenching perspiration and disturbed sleep. Although they are associated with low levels of oestrogen (the oestrogen level rises at ovulation) and therefore indicate a day of infertility, they are not a reliable guide to the end of fertility.

• Changes in other familiar signs of ovulation such as the feeling of fullness around the vagina at the time of ovulation, or abdominal pain associated with ovulation, may disappear. This suggests ovulation is not occurring.

• Recent weight gain. This is commonly associated with declining fertility; but it may be exaggerated by emotional factors such as depression and lethargy, leading to over-eating.

• Changes in the physical characteristics of the cervical mucus. An infertile mucus pattern or dry days increasingly replaces fertile-type mucus. Women who know the Ovulation Method say 'The Peak is not as clear as it was'. This is to be expected and is not a reason to look for a back-up method of contraception. It is now that you learn to recognize your *infertility*.

The mucus during the menopause

You may experience dry days for weeks or months, or scanty amounts of dense mucus which does not change. Typically, the pre-menopausal mucus pattern indicates infertility by *remaining unchanged day after day.*

In some women the mucus is sparse or non-existent, producing a dry sensation. Or it may be crumbly, cloudy, yellow, flaky, clotty, claggy, or even watery and continuous, without ever developing the lubricative qualities of fertile-type mucus. Every woman experiences an individual pattern of infertility which she can learn to recognize.

It is common for dry days to increase in number, and for whole cycles or months to pass during which no mucus is seen or felt. Any return of possible fertility will be mirrored by your mucus. If you are fertile, the fertile-type mucus will be evident by the sensation it produces and your observations of it.

Learning to recognize infertility – keeping a mucus record

The first step is to keep a daily record of your mucus pattern for about a month, avoiding intercourse and genital contact during this time. This ensures that your mucus pattern is not obscured by seminal fluid or vaginal secretions associated with intercourse.

It is not necessary to wait for menstruation before beginning your chart. You may never have another period.

A chart of a woman approaching the menopause is illustrated on p. 119. Don't be disturbed if a mucus pattern typical of a fertile cycle is not apparent. Your pattern is more likely to indicate infertility. Don't wait for the Peak symptom. There may never be one. Simply record your sensations and what you see in your own words; an Ovulation Method teacher will help you interpret the pattern if need be.

If you are infertile, you will soon learn to recognize your own characteristic infertile pattern; and if you are fertile you will learn to recognize your Peak of fertility (p. 43). Be alert for any *change* in your mucus, which will signal the possibility of fertility.

A month after beginning your chart you will be able to apply the Ovulation Method guidelines whether or not you have menstruated, and whether you are fertile or infertile.

Some couples who marry late in their reproductive lives may wish to have a family. As a woman's fertility declines steeply after forty, she will need to observe her pattern very carefully in order to make use of her most fertile days, thereby maximizing her chances of conceiving.

Guidelines for avoiding a pregnancy

These cover all cycle variations of the pre-menopausal period, and are the same guidelines that apply to other phases of your reproductive life. (For a more complete explanation of the guidelines see p. 42.)

MENSTRUATION   During menstruation, avoid intercourse and all genital contact on days of heavy bleeding (in case the menstrual blood obscures the mucus which may occur early in very short cycles). If you do not recognize fertile-type mucus and a Peak prior to menstruation avoid intercourse for three days following bleeding.

THE BASIC INFERTILE PATTERN   During dry days or days of your characteristic infertile-type mucus, use alternate nights for intercourse.

THE CHANGE   On all days of spotty bleeding or mucus that differs from your characteristic infertile pattern avoid intercourse then, and for three days afterwards.

FERTILE-TYPE MUCUS AND THE PEAK   After you recognize fertile-type mucus and the Peak, allow a gap of three days after the Peak before resuming intercourse. The combined fertility of you and your partner is then zero, and intercourse day or night until your next menstruation, carries no possibility of a pregnancy.

Other fertility control methods during the menopause

THE PILL   Evidence that the Pill can cause serious disorders among women approaching the menopause is now well-established. Studies show that the risk of heart and blood vessel disease increases markedly with age among Pill-users (see p. 148). The longer you use the Pill, the more likely are side-effects.

With the onset of infertility, the fertile mucus disappears. However this signal of infertility will not be apparent to you if you use the Pill, because the Pill obscures the normal mucus pattern. Unless you are aware of your mucus pattern, you may take the Pill unnecessarily for many years, putting your health at risk. You will not know when you no longer need the Pill unless you stop taking it and chart the mucus pattern. *This is the only way of finding out if you are infertile.*

THE INTRA-UTERINE DEVICE   Medical authorities advise against an IUD particularly if any of the following conditions are present:
• Abnormal uterine bleeding. IUDs are associated with heavy bleeding and so can worsen this condition.
• Fibroids of the uterus. Fibroids often cause excessive bleeding and an IUD can aggravate this blood loss.
• Diseases affecting the valves of the heart. Damaged heart valves can become infected via the bloodstream following intra-uterine infection from the use of an IUD.
• Past or present pelvic infection. One of the biggest problems with IUDs is that they may introduce infections into the reproductive system. The risk of such an infection is estimated to be three times higher overall in IUD-users than in non-users.[2] Women who have not had children appear to be particularly prone to infection.

STERILIZATION, TUBAL LIGATION AND HYSTERECTOMY
The most common problem following sterilization by tying or burning the Fallopian tubes is prolonged heavy bleeding. Various studies indicate that this complication occurs in 8 to 25 per cent of cases, a situation which may necessitate a hysterectomy. This operation is, of course, a life-saving procedure for some women (for example, if cancer is present). But it should not be undertaken without good reason. Following a hysterectomy, post-operative depression and sexual

dysfunction can occur, often involving loss of libido and pain with intercourse, and the fear of loss of femininity.[3]

Ectopic pregnancy is a well-known complication of tubal ligation.

RHYTHM AND TEMPERATURE METHODS Both these methods have proved unsatisfactory at the time of menopause.

In a study of ninety-eight pre-menopausal women using the Rhythm Method, seventeen became pregnant at the onset of irregularity.[4] This is because the Rhythm Method depends on cycles being approximately constant in length, or remaining within a range that has been established during nine to twelve months' observation. When cycle durations vary markedly – such as when approaching the menopause – arithmetical calculations of ovulation are bound to fail.

The Temperature Method, which relies on a rise in temperature around the time of ovulation, is also unsatisfactory. This is because ovulation occurs less and less frequently as fertility declines at the menopause. Consequently temperature rises are few and far between and couples may wait needlessly for months or even years for the rise in temperature that signals that ovulation has passed. This is most unsatisfactory for relationships and may engender much unhappiness and confusion.

It is extremely frustrating for couples to realize only in retrospect that a long cycle was infertile – and that they have abstained unnecessarily throughout it.

In such a situation they may decide to 'take a chance', with the possibility of an unintended pregnancy. The advantage of the Ovulation Method in this situation is that it enables positive recognition of infertility.

Oestrogen Replacement Therapy

Around the time of the menopause, synthetic oestrogens are often given to replace natural oestrogens which the ovaries are no longer producing at pre-menopausal levels. This treatment should not be considered too soon.

The fall in output of natural oestrogens may be accompanied by emotional disturbances, increased frequency and discomfort of urination, vaginal infections, severe hot flushes, itchiness, vaginal dryness leading to painful intercourse, and bone fragility.

About 25 per cent of women seek some medical help at this time and require knowledgeable and sympathetic management of their problems.[5] Hormone replacement therapy should be carefully considered, for not all symptoms are due to low oestrogens, and even those that are, occur intermittently when the level of oestrogens rises and falls naturally, sometimes for years past the menopause. This is one reason why it is advisable to defer the treatment until well after the menopause, and then to use it only if symptoms are severe and after thorough hormonal assessments are made.

Although oestrogen therapy alleviates some menopausal symptoms, it carries certain risks. These appear to increase if the treatment continues for longer than six months. The risks include endometrial cancer. Various studies suggest that the incidence of this cancer is increased four to eight times in women undergoing prolonged oestrogen hormone therapy without added progestogens.[6, 7]

The trend in hormone treatment at the menopause is to alternate synthetic oestrogen and progestogen (a synthetic substance with similar properties to the naturally occurring hormone, progesterone) thus inducing menstruation every month or two. The purpose of this procedure is to prevent excessive and prolonged build-up of the endometrium. The intermittent removal of the endometrium is a precaution against the increased risk of endometrial cancer which appears to be associated with the use of oestrogen alone. However, synthetic progestogen has its own side-effects including uterine bleeding.

Other possible side-effects of hormone replacement therapy include breast cancer, gall bladder disease, disorders of blood vessels, severe headaches (believed to be caused by the progestogen), rapid weight gain, and troublesome, uncontrolled uterine bleeding.[8] Frequent heavy bleeding may lead to anaemia, and subsequent tiredness and depression. Investigation may be required and possibly a curettage or a biopsy of uterine tissue.

When synthetic oestrogens are taken, the mucus pattern is disturbed (synthetic hormones – by influencing centres in the brain – suppress natural hormones); the cervix produces a continuous discharge which resembles fertile-type mucus and may be blood-stained. So, if you are using the Ovulation Method, such treatment will result in unnecessary abstinence.

Progestogen at the menopause

Progestogen (often in the form of the Pill) is sometimes prescribed to pre-menopausal women to make their cycles more of average length by prolonging the post-ovulatory phase (which tends to become shorter as fertility declines). However this treatment is inadvisable for a number of reasons.

By a disturbance of the main pituitary ovarian interaction, ovulation is often abolished. Progestogen when used to prolong the cycle length alters the normal development of the endometrium and can cause erratic uncontrollable bleeding. In the unlikely event of implantation occurring, there is a risk of damage to the foetus. The progestogen alters the mucus produced by the cervix, making assessment of fertility virtually impossible.

By acting on the bone marrow cells which are involved in blood clotting, progestogen may result in the production of numerous small clots which may block blood vessels in the brain causing severe headaches. These small clots may also settle in the bones, causing areas of bone death,[9] and give rise to pain in the limbs. Larger clots settling in vital blood vessels may result in strokes, blindness and heart disease.

Alternatives to hormone therapy

It is worth pursuing alternatives to hormone therapy, because they do not alter the body's chemistry.

If a woman is happy and content, natural lubrication of the vagina will occur prior to lovemaking. Her partner needs to know this and take time in lovemaking. Then it is unnecessary to use lubricative creams or jellies, or oestrogen creams, all of which disturb the pattern of natural secretions. It is easy to set up a vicious circle: a dry vagina makes intercourse painful – painful intercourse is resisted – this leads to disharmony and prevents the flow of natural secretions in the vagina.

Sympathetic counselling is often necessary to identify problems which have nothing to do with the menopause but which, by causing anxiety and distress, may worsen menopausal symptoms.

Increased efforts to improve communication between partners can help. Husbands benefit greatly from an explanation of the climacteric.

Rest each day and attention to general health are important. A woman at this time tends to become much less active. It is most important that regular exercise is taken; healthy muscles help maintain joints and bones in good condition.

Following the menopause, if severe physical symptoms – such as urinary discomfort and constant itching – persist, oestrogen replacement therapy in small doses should be considered. Local oestrogen creams may prove valuable.

The problem of osteoporosis (a weakness of the bone structure), which is associated with stress-related hormones interacting with low levels of female sex hormones, occurs in some women after the menopause. Clinical research is continuing in order to establish whether oestrogens are of any value in its control.

Hot flushes are usually of nuisance value and do not warrant the giving of oestrogens except in circumstances of unusual severity. They do not always respond to oestrogens and there are alternative remedies. Clonidine hydrochloride, a non-hormonal medication, is effective sometimes. It is natural for a woman to lose her hot flushes for several weeks at a time without treatment.

The cervical mucus and your gynaecological health

Once you can recognize your normal mucus pattern, any significant deviation – such as blood-stained or profuse mucus – indicates the need for a medical examination.

Any unusual bleeding should also be investigated and a satisfactory explanation provided.

Natural irregular bleeding can be explained by knowing the mucus pattern. This can spare a woman unnecessary curettage. Early diagnosis of disorders offers the best prospect of a successful treatment.

If all examinations and investigations prove normal and you are not taking synthetic hormones (as explained, these confuse diagnosis by causing uterine bleeding and mucus changes), charting may indicate that the mucus pattern you are now observing signifies a new situation of infertility.

'For the past five years – since I was forty-three – my menstrual cycles have been irregular. At the beginning of this time I was using the Temperature Method.

The length of my cycles was sometimes sixty days, and in some cases there was no temperature rise, indicating that I was not always ovulating.

When ovulation did occur, I was using the post-ovulatory days for intercourse as well as the days of my menstrual bleeding.

My last child – now aged two – resulted from intercourse on the first day of bleeding after a long cycle; the bleeding was in fact associated with ovulation rather than the start of my menstrual period.

After the birth of this child, my husband and I were advised to abstain from intercourse for six months. We were told that if no menstrual period occurred during that time, I could assume that I was permanently infertile. Surely there was a better way. I then consulted an obstetrician who prescribed Norethisterone – a synthetic form of the hormone progesterone. The aim of this medication was to produce cycles of a regular length, so that I could use the Rhythm Method with temperature as a guide to fertile cycles. However, I did not bleed for six months, and then experienced a series of very heavy losses. I next developed headaches, pain in my arms and legs, and naturally enough, considerable anxiety. Everything was going wrong – including my marriage.

At this time, I heard about the Ovulation Method. Although sceptical, I sought the advice of a local Ovulation Method teacher.

My first chart after stopping Norethisterone, indicated a Basic Infertile Pattern of unchanging, sticky mucus. It was not difficult to convince me to follow the Early Day Rule (intercourse on alternate nights) while the Basic Infertile Pattern continued. After a few patches of fertile-type mucus, my pattern settled down to a constant infertile pattern, and I knew that I could safely put all worries about a pregnancy behind me.'

Every woman must make decisions about how to control her fertility as the menopause approaches. For some readers, the menopause is imminent; for others, it will occur some time in the future. Whatever your age, you will benefit from learning your signs of fertility and infertility now. It is not difficult to learn the method even when you are mostly infertile.

If you are in a dilemma – not knowing when to stop the Pill, or if you think sterilization is the only way – don't despair. Remember, after one month of charting, most women can recognize the days when intercourse will not result in pregnancy.

An understanding of the physiological and emotional accompaniments of declining fertility will explain many doubts, protect your health, and may open the way to improved relationships with family members.

12

Difficulties in conceiving

Approximately 15 per cent of couples trying to have a child are unable to do so.[1] Another 10 per cent have fewer children than they desire. Yet most couples are totally unprepared for infertility and unaware that in many cases it can be overcome.

Infertility may produce many unexpected feelings – isolation, helplessness, guilt, anger, despair, and grief for the child not born. It may be the cause of mutual accusations, and create demands on partners, family, and friends, whose support and advice is sought.

However, the advice given is not always accurate or sympathetic. And unless it is scientifically well-founded, suggestions about how to overcome an infertility problem can further damage an already disturbed relationship. So it is important to seek doctors or counsellors who are knowledgeable in this field.

Infertility is usually defined as the inability to conceive after twelve to eighteen months of sexual intercourse without contraception.

The ability to conceive and give birth reaches its peak at about the age of twenty-five in both men and women. In women, reproductive ability declines between thirty and forty, then very rapidly as the menopause approaches. In men fertility gradually diminishes from about the age of fifty.[2]

Many couples wanting a child who seek the help of a doctor will eventually conceive and give birth. They may have become unnecessarily alarmed at the delay in achieving a pregnancy. In many cases all that is needed is reassurance, provided by discussing the processes involved in reproduction and emphasizing that intercourse without contraception does

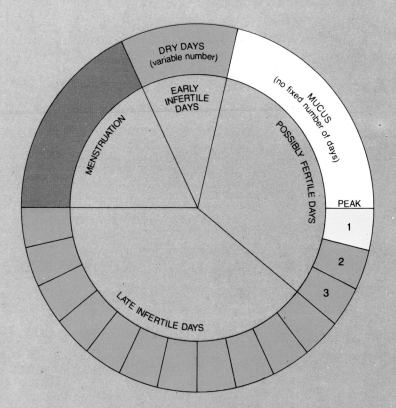

THE MENSTRUAL CYCLE
The mucus pattern of fertility and infertility

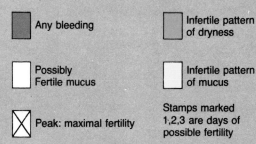

COLOUR CODE FOR CHARTS

Any bleeding

Infertile pattern
of dryness

Possibly
Fertile mucus

Infertile pattern
of mucus

Peak: maximal fertility

Stamps marked
1,2,3 are days of
possible fertility

CHARTING: SOME COMMON EXAMPLES

Figure 1(a) FIRST RECORD OF A CYCLE. Record what you see and feel: red – bleeding; green – dryness; white – any mucus. Try to identify the Peak (X).

Figure 1(b) Record with a yellow stamp, mucus after the Peak.

Figure 1(c) Refer to chapter 6 where the guidelines are explained.

Figure 2 A SHORT CYCLE with the Peak on Day 5. Intercourse should be avoided on all days of bleeding because ovulation may occur early.

Figure 3 A LONG CYCLE with the Peak on Day 23. Careful charting after the supposed Peak (Day 21) is necessary because occasionally fertile characteristics return (Day 23).

Figure 4 THE EFFECT OF INTERCOURSE ON THE MUCUS. Note the effect of seminal fluid on the day following intercourse, and application of the Early Day Rules (chapter 6). From three days past the Peak, all days are available for intercourse.

Figure 1(a) First record of cycle

Figure 1(b) Same chart stamped for correct record of fertile and infertile mucus

Figure 1(c) Applying the guidelines to the cycle

Figure 2 A short cycle

Figure 3 A long cycle

Figure 4 The effect of intercourse on the mucus

Figure 5 Continuous mucus

Figure 6(a) An infertile cycle

Figure 6(b) An infertile cycle

Figure 7 Pregnancy achieved

Figure 8 A stress cycle

Figure 5 CONTINUOUS MUCUS. When mucus is continuous, several cycles may be necessary to identify the point of change from infertile to fertile mucus. In this cycle a change in sensation (Day 8) marked the start of the fertile phase.

Figure 6(a) and 6(b) TWO INFERTILE CYCLES. Hormone analysis confirmed ovulation (Day 14/15) in both cycles but intercourse at this time did not result in conception for either woman. No mucus occurred in 6(a) and in 6(b) mucus was present but lacked fertile characteristics.

Figure 7 PREGNANCY ACHIEVED. The use of alternate days for intercourse enabled this couple to recognize the beginning of the fertile phase. (This is important if mucus is sparse.) The couple then used several days for intercourse to achieve a pregnancy.

Figure 8 A STRESS CYCLE. Stress on Day 9 alerted this woman to the possibility that ovulation might be delayed. The couple applied the Early Day Rules for the whole cycle because no clear Peak was recorded.

Figure 9 Cycles showing return to fertility after the Pill

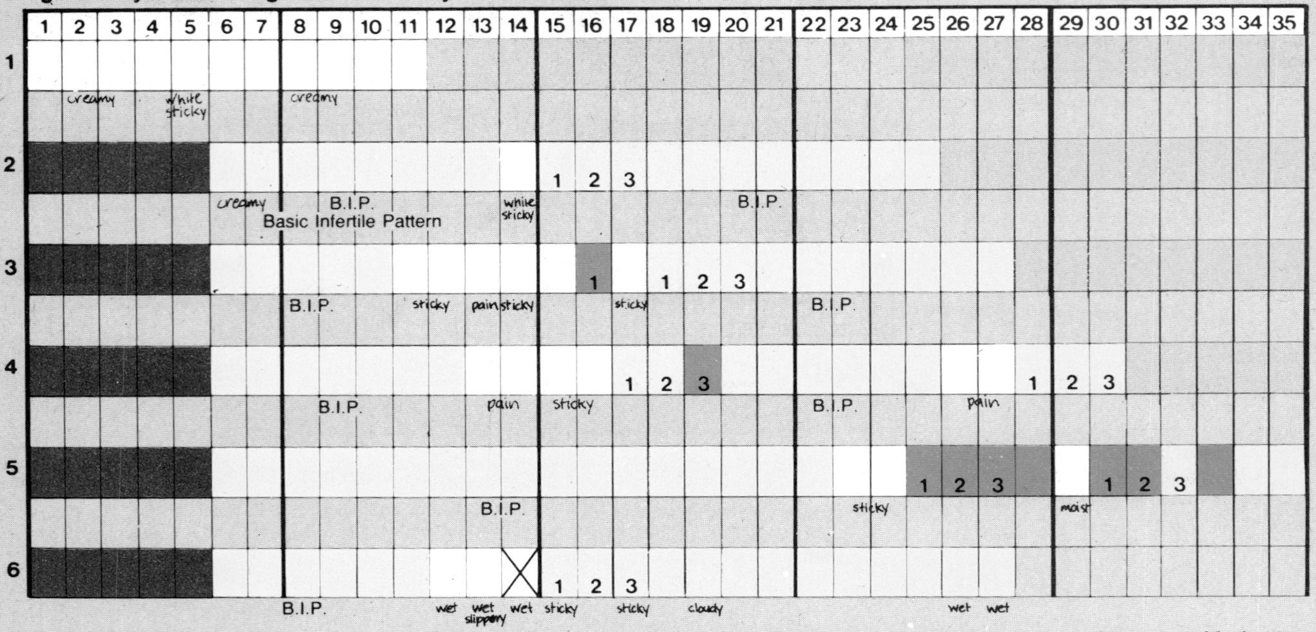

Chart grid, days 1–35 across the top, cycles 1–6 down the side.

Cycle	Recorded observations (by day)
1	creamy (2–3); white sticky (4–5); creamy (7); creamy (8)
2	creamy (6–7); B.I.P. Basic Infertile Pattern (8–9); white sticky (13–14); 1 2 3 (15–17)
3	B.I.P. (8–9); sticky (11); sticky (12); pain/sticky (13); 1 (16); sticky (17); 1 2 3 (18–20); B.I.P. (21)
4	B.I.P. (8–9); pain (13); sticky (15); 1 (16); 1 2 3 (17–19); B.I.P. (22); B.I.P. (22); pain (27); 1 (28); 2 3 (29–30)
5	B.I.P. (8–9); B.I.P. (13); B.I.P. (22); sticky (24); 1 2 3 (25–27); pain (27); wet wet (26); moist (29); 1 2 3 (29–31); 3 (32)
6	B.I.P. (8); X (14); 1 2 3 (15–17)

Bottom annotations: wet wet wet slippery / wet wet sticky / sticky sticky / cloudy / wet wet / moist

Figure 9 AFTER COMING OFF THE PILL. In her first learning chart, this woman recorded her observations of mucus with white stamps. After her first bleed she could recognize her Basic Infertile Pattern of mucus (see chapter 6) and marked these days with yellow stamps. She then used white stamps to indicate possible fertility when any change in the mucus was apparent. She ovulated in the last cycle.

Figure 10 Disturbance to normal cycle due to an ovarian cyst

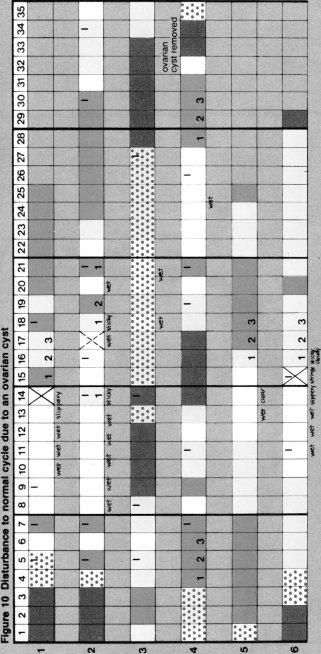

Figure 10 AN ABNORMAL CYCLE – an ovarian cyst. The first line shows this woman's normal pattern. Then a long cycle occurred (lines 2 to 4), complicated by blood-spotting, an abnormal mucus pattern, and bleeding that she recognized as different from her normal menstrual flow. Such a change from her normal cycle alerted this woman to seek medical advice. An ovarian cyst was diagnosed and then removed (line 4). The pattern improved immediately, yet no Peak was recognized in the next cycle. Although a possibly fertile pattern was recorded in the last cycle, the return of fertility was delayed until the following cycle when pregnancy was achieved as desired.

Figure 11 Breastfeeding

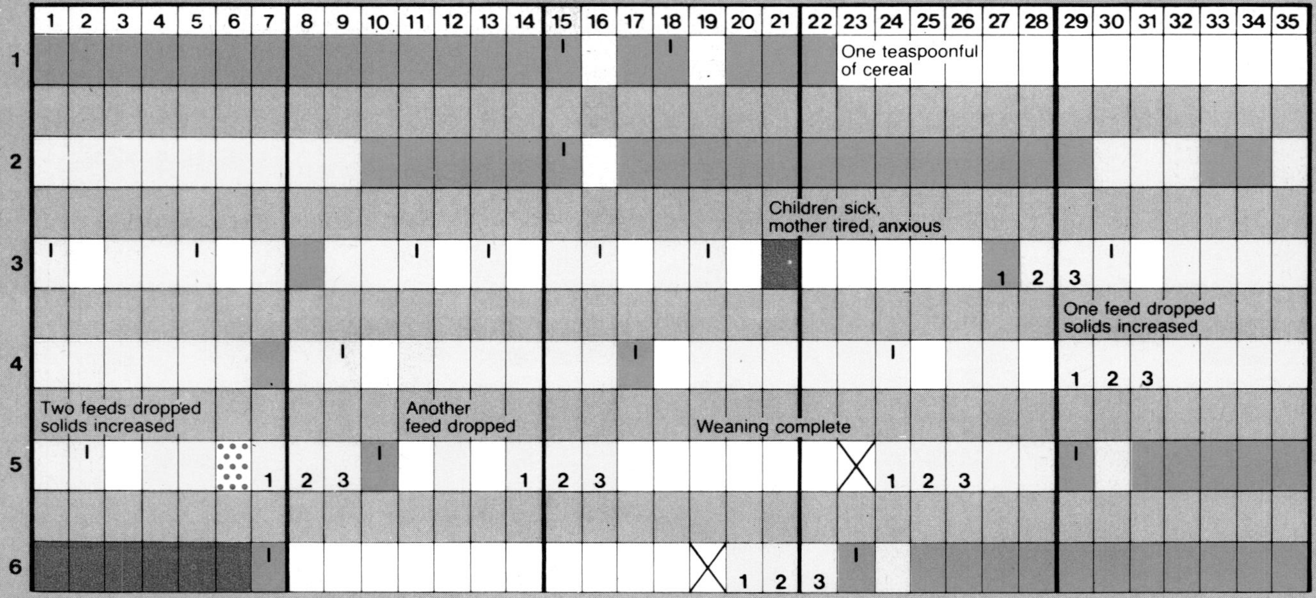

Figure 11 BREASTFEEDING. This is the chart of a woman who learned the method while breastfeeding her three-month-old baby. Two weeks charting without intercourse was sufficient to determine a continuing pattern of dryness (green stamp). Mucus with unchanging characteristics was recorded with a yellow stamp. All days following intercourse were recorded with a white stamp.

When the pattern changed (line 3) with bleeding and five days of fertile-type mucus, intercourse was deferred until three days after the return of the Basic Infertile Pattern. The Peak was recognized (line 5), indicating the return of fertility. (See chapter 10 for the method guidelines during breastfeeding.)

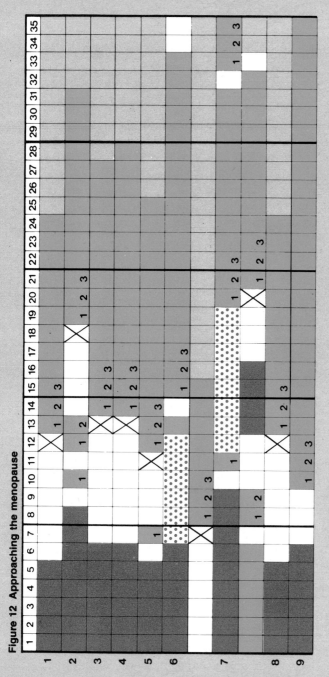

Figure 12 Approaching the menopause

Figure 12 APPROACHING THE MENOPAUSE. When approaching the menopause a woman's normal pattern changes, leading to eventual infertility. This woman experienced irregularity, prolonged menstrual bleeding (cycles 6 and 7), a short interval between the Peak and menstruation (cycle 6) and pre-ovulatory bleeding (cycle 7). By following the method guidelines outlined in chapters 6 and 11, this woman was able to assess her infertile and possibly fertile days. Following cycle 9 she recognized continuing infertility.

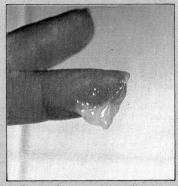

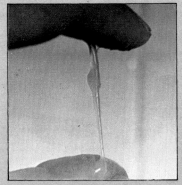

1. Pre-ovulatory mucus will not stretch, and breaks

2. Fertile-type stretchy mucus

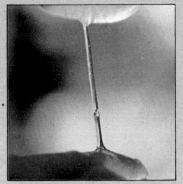

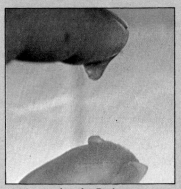

3. Clear fertile-type mucus close to the Peak

4. Mucus after the Peak

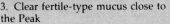

THE KEY TO FERTILITY CONTROL: THE MUCUS

The photographs above show examples of one woman's mucus. Your own mucus may not look quite like this but you will quickly come to recognize what is fertile and what is infertile.

The lubricative sensation which indicates high fertility may persist for a day or two after the mucus is no longer visible.

The mucus and the guidelines for the method are described in chapters 4, 5 and 6.

not guarantee an immediate pregnancy. Studies indicate that in those trying to conceive, fewer than a third will achieve their goal within the first month, only 50 per cent by six months, and 80 to 90 per cent by eighteen months.[3]

Advice about timing intercourse to coincide with ovulation often proves invaluable. Some women produce the fertile-type mucus, essential if sperm are to reach the egg and maintain their fertilizing capacity for only a day or two around the time of ovulation and only in some cycles. The Ovulation Method enables you to recognize this time of fertility and maximize your chances of conception occurring. Intercourse when you recognize fertile-type mucus provides the maximum chance of conception. This simple information has helped many couples to conceive.

A temperature rise will provide confirmatory evidence of ovulation. However, it will be of no use in helping you time intercourse to coincide with ovulation since it usually occurs one to two days after ovulation (range four days before to six days after ovulation) by which time the egg is dead.

Causes of infertility

Infertility may be a temporary or a permanent problem, and should be viewed as the problem of a couple rather than of an individual even when the major component of the problem rests with one partner. Various studies indicate that in about 30 per cent of cases, male factors are mainly responsible; while the main problem lies with the female partner in about 45 per cent of cases.

In the remainder, no cause of the infertility can be found, and contributory factors from both partners may be involved. Although the chances of achieving a pregnancy when the cause of infertility is unknown are often quoted as only 20 per cent, skilful counselling can increase the success rate substantially.

As new techniques of assessing infertility become available, and as we improve our understanding of the psychological, as well as the physical aspects of the problem, success rates are improving. Today, for example, an estimated 60 per cent of women with disorders of ovulation can be helped to become natural parents.[4]

In this chapter we shall concentrate on some of the common causes of sub-fertility and infertility that can be helped by an awareness of the mucus. With many causes, the cervical mucus provides the first indication that all is not well. When treatment is successful, the mucus again acts as a signal – this time indicating the return of fertility.

The Ovulation Method and infertility

The clinical and experimental studies on the cervical mucus that provide the basis of the Ovulation Method have proved invaluable in the treatment of infertility.

Recognition of fertile-type mucus, coupled with the correct timing of intercourse to coincide with the Peak, have proved to be important factors in the improved management of infertility in recent years.

When you know that ovulation is imminent by observing your mucus signals, you have the knowledge to greatly increase your chances of conception. (See p. 39 for a description of the mucus signs.)

In some couples, suitable conditions for achieving a pregnancy – including the presence of mucus capable of supporting and assisting transport of the sperm cells – occur in only a few cycles each year, and perhaps for half a day only in each cycle. If you are having difficulty conceiving, you will need to be particularly watchful for these occasions.

'At first I thought I wasn't producing any mucus. Then, one day, after keeping watch for six months, I saw it. There was no doubt in my mind. We used that day for intercourse. The next day the fertile mucus was gone. Six weeks later doctors confirmed that our baby was on the way.'

But no amount of Ovulation Method knowledge can restore function to obstructed Fallopian tubes or remove cysts from ovaries, or rectify damage to the testes that is affecting sperm production. The Ovulation Method is not the answer to every infertility problem, and it would be quite wrong to delay a full medical investigation due to an exaggerated idea of what can be achieved by using the method. Once an underlying physical problem, such as blocked tubes, is rectified, the Ovulation Method can be used to advantage.

Increasingly, doctors who deal with infertility problems are recognizing the value of the mucus signals, and are referring couples for skilled Ovulation Method tuition while they proceed with their independent investigations.

Competent teaching, backed by encouragement and the opportunity to discuss the mucus signals and their relationship to reproduction, is vital.

The importance of correct information

Incorrect information can contribute to apparent infertility. Some women, unaware of the significance of the fertile mucus, have believed it to be a sign of infection which could be transmitted to their partner. As a result, they have avoided intercourse at this, their most fertile time.

Others have been embarrassed by the profusion of the fertile-type mucus and, not recognizing its importance, have likewise deferred intercourse. Attempts to remove it with douches and creams may have rendered the environment of the vagina hostile to sperm, contributing to an infertility problem.

Some couples try complicated and unnecessary techniques to achieve a pregnancy. They may, for example, have intercourse daily, which can prove counter-productive. For while some men can maintain a high quality of semen production with frequent – even daily – intercourse, others cannot.

Where frequent intercourse has occurred during the fertile phase of the cycle without a pregnancy resulting, it is likely that a rest from intercourse for a few days before the most fertile mucus appears, will prove beneficial.

Factors involved in conception

The achievement of a pregnancy involves a complex chain of events. The egg cell must be healthy and must find its way from the ovary into the Fallopian tube. Healthy sperm cells must arrive in the vagina at a time when the cervical mucus is able to nourish and channel them through the uterus. The sperm passage along the Fallopian tube, assisted by the muscular movements of the uterus and tubes, must not be obstructed. Once fertilization has occurred, the developing egg (zygote) must travel back through the tube to the uterus, arriving when both it, and the uterine lining, are at a suitable stage of development for implantation.

Precise timing and optimal conditions are crucial in a number of these events. And the disturbance of any one of the delicate physiological processes may make pregnancy difficult or even impossible to achieve. Many influences can tip the balance, including correct information and psychological factors.

During initial investigations, it usually becomes clear whether the basic problem is physical or psychological and, if the latter, whether time and reassurance will help.

Psychological factors: anxiety, tension

The investigation and management of infertility can itself stress couples, and it is not surprising that this can increase anxiety, which in turn can affect fertility.

Couples seeking help may be shy and anxious. The virility of the man and the femininity of the woman may seem to be in question, and investigations may loom large and threatening.

The fact that pregnancy often occurs when stress is taken out of the situation indicates how important psychological factors can be. An indication of their importance is the finding that 30 per cent of women undergoing artificial insemination fail to ovulate, or ovulate poorly during the stresses of the treatment period, after previously ovulating normally.[5]

'After trying to have a child for six years without success, my husband and I decided to adopt a baby. Within six months I was pregnant. We can only conclude that our anxiety about conceiving somehow obstructed the normal course of events.'

Fatigue is sometimes a contributory factor to fertility problems. And a rest from work may provide the 'cure'. Undue stress from overwork or emotional distress is associated with lowered fertility in both men and women.

When the problem of infertility becomes an overriding concern, it is not uncommon for a woman to feel she is regarded as a producer rather than as a woman loved just for herself. It is a mistake to assume that 'everything will be all right if we can have a child'. When partners become totally important to each other 'no matter what', conception may happen unexpectedly – as though the baby had been waiting.

'Things were getting really bad. I had so many tests and so had Phil. I had kept a chart for eight months and everybody said we were normal . . . The best thing you told me after teaching me about the mucus was to forget the chart and concentrate on our life together. I gave up work, took some cooking lessons, pampered us both a bit and it happened. I really knew I was fertile. When I relaxed so did our love-making – and it became natural, not an exercise.'

Sometimes apparent infertility occurs when communication between partners breaks down. This may be reflected in a nervous sensitivity when one touches the other. This tension may prove a barrier to conception.

In such cases as this, conscious efforts by both partners to show a loving and caring attitude without looking for sexual rewards can help greatly.

Psychological factors can operate to produce a painful spasm of the vagina called vaginismus, or an inhibition of the secretions that normally lubricate the vagina. Both these conditions make intercourse difficult and emotionally distressing for both partners, and this may affect fertility.

Even normal functioning of the Fallopian tubes may be disturbed by anxiety.

On the male side, psychological influences can contribute to impotence, where an erection cannot be maintained adequately to allow successful vaginal penetration leading to orgasm and ejaculation. Highly specialized counselling may be warranted.

When both partners are involved in seeking a solution, lasting benefits are more likely. And when good information is available, couples themselves make the best counsellors. In the event where the problem of infertility cannot be overcome, working through the situation together often produces a strengthening of a relationship and an unbreakable bond of mutual love and support.

Investigations

Early investigation of infertility should involve both partners. It should include:

• A medical history of both partners including sexual development, past contraceptive usage, tuberculosis or pelvic inflammatory disease, stress situations, excessive tiredness, weight problems, and venereal disease.

• Physical examination of both partners including a complete gynaecological examination of the woman.

• Charting the menstrual cycle according to the Ovulation Method. The cervical mucus pattern will provide information about some of the essentials of fertility. It also provides information about a woman's gynaecological health which may help unravel the infertility problem. For instance, disturbance of the mucus pattern may suggest the presence of infection, ovarian cysts, endometriosis or other abnormalities, particularly of the cervix. A hormonal disturbance may be suspected in the absence of fertile mucus and will require investigation.

Further investigations include an assessment of hormone levels, a Huhner's (post-coital) test, a hysterosalpingogram, and laparoscopy.

HORMONE ASSESSMENT   The procedure followed depends on the symptoms of the fertility problem. In the absence of a recognizable mucus pattern, the hormones from the ovaries are studied. These and further investigations require the attention of a specialist.

HUHNER'S TEST   This test involves the collection of a mucus sample from the cervix about four to twelve hours after intercourse around the time of your Peak fertility, as judged by the mucus. A semen analysis is made by studying the number, activity and form of sperm cells under high magnification.

The great value of the Huhner's test is that it assesses the compatibility of your partner's sperm with your fertile-type mucus, and confirms that intercourse has successfully deposited sperm cells in the vagina.

The test must be timed to coincide with the fertile mucus near or at the Peak of fertility, since the sperm cells die promptly in an unfavourable mucus environment.

The Huhner's test may indicate compatible sperm-mucus interaction, or it may suggest disorders of sperm production, cervical or vaginal infections, hostile mucus at the time of ovulation, or – very rarely – the presence of sperm antibodies which destroy or damage the sperm.

HYSTEROSALPINGOGRAM   A hysterosalpingogram involves taking X-ray pictures of the reproductive organs while a radiopaque dye is injected through the vagina into the Fallopian tubes. This helps to determine whether the tubes are closed off, for example by scar tissue or following an inflammation which has caused the tubal lining to adhere in places.

The hysterosalpingogram shows the shape of the uterine cavity, the state of each tube, and the site of an obstruction, if any. Such obstruction may be suspected following any pelvic or abdominal infection.

Sometimes, performing a hysterosalpingogram will clear the Fallopian tubes of minor obstruction and a pregnancy may follow soon afterwards.

LAPAROSCOPY   Doctors may use the techniques of laparoscopy or culdoscopy to check that the Fallopian tubes are open and to investigate physical abnormalities, such as ovarian cysts, fibroids of the uterus, or tubal adhesions which may be affecting your fertility. These procedures involve introducing a telescope-like instrument either through the abdominal wall or the vaginal wall to directly observe the internal organs. A dye may also be introduced during laparoscopy to enable assessment of the internal organs.

Physical causes of infertility

Although far more is known about infertility in women than men, there are still great gaps in our knowledge, so that in a significant proportion of women, despite extensive and sophisticated efforts, the cause of infertility remains obscure.

The congenital abnormalities of the reproductive tract and chromosomal abnormalities are generally considered as rare causes of infertility.

More common are the endocrine causes, such as deficient production of certain hormones by the pituitary gland (Follicle Stimulating Hormone and Luteinizing Hormone); excessive production by the pituitary of the hormone stimulating breast-milk production (prolactin); deficient progesterone production by the ovary; and other less specific and less well understood hormonal mechanisms.
– *World Health*, Journal of the World Health Organization, September 1978, 30–33.

In women, it is estimated that abnormalities of the Fallopian tubes are the cause of about 25 per cent of infertility problems, disorders of the ovaries and of ovulation account for about 10 per cent of cases, and other identifiable causes about 10 per cent.[6]

Often no major abnormality can be found to account for the infertility problem. Current research however shows that infections of the reproductive organs increasingly are implicated. Although these are often symptomless, they can cause significant damage.

Tubal abnormalities

This is the most common identifiable cause of infertility, and is often difficult to correct.

The Fallopian tubes are particularly vulnerable to infection, and any scarring or destruction of the delicate tube lining may affect the passage of the sperm or egg, making conception impossible. If the microscopic hairs lining the tubes – so vital to sperm and egg movement – are damaged, this may disrupt the synchronization necessary for implantation of the developing egg in the nutritive endometrium. In humans this mutual suitability of uterus and the fertilized egg exists for only about thirty-six hours.

Likewise, the muscular lining of the tubes which is partially responsible for sperm and egg movement must be in good condition. If movement along the tube is too slow, the zygote may implant and develop within the tube, resulting in an ectopic pregnancy. This carries an increased risk of rupture and destruction of the tube, loss of the foetus, and reduced fertility (since only one Fallopian tube will then be functioning). Or if movement along the tube is too fast, the developing egg can be hurried into the uterus before the imbedding site is ready to accept it. Hormones control this time-sensitive mechanism and synthetic hormones can disrupt it.

DIAGNOSIS AND TREATMENT   What if both partners are in good health and charting of the mucus indicates a normal pattern, yet conception fails to occur after intercourse during the fertile phase of two to three cycles? The next step is to do a Huhner's test and to check that the Fallopian tubes are not blocked by performing a hysterosalpingogram or laparoscopy, or both.

A medical history may suggest how damage to the delicate hair-lined channel or muscle walls of the tubes has occurred. Possible causes include infections, surgery, a ruptured appendix, tuberculosis, venereal disease especially gonorrhoea, as well as other pelvic infections.[7]

Adhesions – bands of fibrous tissue which may develop following inflammation or surgery – may require surgical removal.

The success of the treatment varies according to the extent of the damage, especially if the fringed ends of the tubes near the ovary (the fimbriae) are involved.

If the cause of the infertility is a previous sterilization

involving burning or tying of the tubes, and a reversal is now sought, this may be possible; however only limited success has been achieved to date.

Problems associated with the ovaries and ovulation

Disorders associated with the ovaries may be suggested by abnormalities of the mucus pattern, or by disturbance of the normal menstrual pattern. (A change in the length of the cycle does not indicate an abnormality.)

Failure to release egg cells may be due to a fault within the ovaries themselves, or to failure of one or both of the hormones released by the pituitary gland (Follicle Stimulating Hormone and Luteinizing Hormone). Urine analysis of hormones can readily furnish information about ovulation. Blood tests are also available.

These hormones in their turn may be deficient due to lack of a 'releasing hormone' from the hypothalamus which triggers their output.

Rarely, the ovaries 'dry-up' prematurely and no egg cells are available. No fertile mucus is produced. This happens to every woman in the months or years before the menopause, which occurs on average about the age of fifty. But every now and then it occurs much earlier and is then called premature ovarian failure. Since no eggs are available for ovulation, nothing can be done to overcome this problem.

Some women have regular monthly periods but do not ovulate (the cycles are then termed anovulatory). On keeping a daily mucus record, it is seen that these cycles lack the Peak mucus signal. Hormonal investigations show a persistently low production of the hormone, progesterone, throughout the cycle, and absence of a basal body temperature rise which is an indicator that ovulation has occurred.

Other women will notice that they have fertile mucus only occasionally, and their cycles may be very irregular. Medical investigation is necessary to determine whether lack of fertile mucus in most cycles is due to a failure to ovulate or an abnormality of the cervix.

Treatment with fertility drugs to induce ovulation often proves successful. The fertility drugs are discussed later in this chapter.

Another ovary-related problem occurs in the situation where the interval between the Peak of fertility and the following menstruation is less than ten days. This is due to a deficiency of the corpus luteum. In this event the endometrium is shed prematurely. Treatment to overcome this premature shedding is available with the hormone Human Chorionic Gonadotrophin (HCG) or Bromocriptine (p. 133).

Sometimes menstruation fails to occur (a condition known as amenorrhoea) and except where the uterus is abnormal, this means that ovulation has failed.

Amenorrhoea is defined as the absence of menstruation for six months or more. Stress, fatigue, psychological disturbances, obesity, weight loss, anorexia nervosa, thyroid disease, diabetes, an abnormal growth of the pituitary gland, or the Pill, are among the causes.

A significant number of women with absent or infrequent bleeding of less than one year's duration, or with amenorrhoea after coming off the Pill, ovulate spontaneously during the investigation period. This may be due to reassurance provided by sympathetic and well-informed counsellors and doctors.

Another possible cause of the amenorrhoea is an excess of the hormone prolactin produced by the pituitary gland in the brain. (Prolactin is the hormone which stimulates breast milk production.) This situation requires skilful medical management to exclude the possibility of a tumour of the pituitary gland. Treatment with the drug Bromocriptine has been successful in achieving a 95 per cent ovulation rate and a 75 per cent conception rate.[8]

A common cause of infertility related to the ovaries is polycystic ovaries. This occurs when both ovaries are enlarged by multiple cysts, resulting in an erratic mucus pattern, lack of a Peak mucus symptom, and intermittent bleeding. A woman who is familiar with her normal mucus pattern can recognize the abnormality at an early stage. Other features which may indicate this condition include a tendency towards hairiness and obesity.

Treatment with the fertility drug, Clomiphene, or successful removal of the cysts, has enabled women with this condition to have children.

DIAGNOSIS AND TREATMENT   Through various tests, your doctor will try to assess at which level the fault lies. These tests may include hormonal analysis of blood or urine samples.

Fertility drugs

In some women, ovulation can be stimulated by the so-called fertility drugs. These include Clomiphene, Bromocriptine, and the Gonadotrophins. They are only useful if the basic problem is failure to ovulate which will be indicated by the absence of fertile mucus and by evaluation of hormone levels. The results of hormone measurements on urine or blood samples will determine which fertility drug – if any – will be useful in treatment.

CLOMIPHENE   This is a synthetic anti-oestrogen which appears to induce ovulation by stimulating the release of Follicle Stimulating Hormone (FSH) and Luteinizing Hormone (LH).

It is often used for women whose fertility has been impaired by the Pill and who wish to have a baby.

Patience is strongly recommended. It is preferable to allow the natural return of fertility, even if this takes two years, rather than to use a drug such as Clomiphene prematurely, for its effects are not yet fully documented. It is known that it reduces mucus production, so that the fertile mucus may be present for only a very short time at ovulation. Therefore anyone on this treatment needs to be particularly alert for the fertile-type mucus.

Ovulation rates of 80 per cent can be achieved with Clomiphene, with pregnancy rates of about 40 per cent.

The low pregnancy rate appears to be due to the dampening

down effect of the Clomiphene on the cervical mucus, which plays an essential role in sperm fertilizing capacity.

BROMOCRIPTINE   This should only be used following a full medical investigation to eliminate the possibility of a pituitary tumour. This drug is useful where excessive production of the hormone prolactin, which stimulates breast-milk production, is blocking the action of hormones involved in ovulation. Bromocriptine switches off the production of prolactin, enabling other hormones to exert an effect.

GONADOTROPHINS   These are the most potent and expensive fertility drugs available and are used when the body's own production of these hormones is insufficient to cause ovulation, for example, after removal of the pituitary gland. The Gonadotrophins are reserved for patients who have not responded to other ovulation-inducing drugs, when the ovary has been shown to be able to respond. They include Human Chorionic Gonadotrophin (HCG), Human Menopausal Gonadotrophin (HMG) and Human Pituitary Gonadotrophin (HPG).

These bypass the hypothalamus and pituitary gland and substitute for the two pituitary hormones, FSH and LH.

The effectiveness of the Gonadotrophins depends on whether the ovaries are capable of being stimulated. Cases have been reported of ovaries dormant for many years, yet responding with full ovulation within ten days of commencing therapy.

Extremely close supervision is essential, since over-stimulation of the ovaries can easily occur, resulting in the rapid development of large ovarian cysts, or in multiple births.

A high ovulation rate of 90 per cent can be achieved under careful supervision. Sixty per cent or more of women treated become pregnant. And 20 per cent of such pregnancies are multiple births, mainly twins.

If the problem is a short post-ovulatory phase of ten days or less (as can be readily seen by charting the mucus pattern),

HCG helps to prevent the premature shedding of the endometrium by providing support for the corpus luteum.

Infections

A woman's fertility may be impaired by pelvic inflammatory disease, a term which refers to infections of the reproduction organs, and particularly those affecting the Fallopian tubes.

The disease may follow procedures such as curettage or the insertion of an IUD or it may be sexually transmitted.[9]

An infection may or may not produce symptoms. Often damage is done before investigations detect the organism responsible. Early treatment is essential.

A multitude of factors may affect the internal environment. Douches, vaginal creams, and sometimes the use of the Pill, create an environment suitable for the growth of certain organisms. Several organisms involved in causing pelvic inflammatory disease may then find their way to the uterus where the presence of an IUD may help them become established.

A recent study shows that the risk of uterine infection in women under the age of thirty with IUDs is five times greater than among non-IUD users.[10] It is thought that the offending IUDs may cause a break in the endometrial surface, thus permitting bacterial invasion of the endometrium and of adjacent blood and lymph vessels.

Another possibility is that some IUDs contain organisms even before they are inserted, and that these produce infection which may be associated with symptoms of irritation, soreness, and a burning sensation when urinating. The mucus may be continuous with an unpleasant odour.

Recent research suggests a very important organism in pelvic inflammatory disease is T-mycoplasma.[11] Mycoplasmas are the smallest free-living organisms known and are intermediate between viruses and bacteria. Antibiotics can clear them up. How mycoplasma infections relate to infertility and foetal loss is still unclear. Some researchers believe that they cause the endometrium to be hostile to the fertilized and developing egg.

Douches and chemicals used in the vagina

Douches, vaginal deodorants, and lubricative jellies have been associated with diminished fertility. These preparations may contain chemicals capable of killing sperm cells, or they may disturb the vaginal environment by causing allergies or inflammatory reactions which impair sperm survival. They also tend to obscure the mucus pattern, making assessment of your fertile phase difficult. They should be discontinued to maximize the chances of a pregnancy occurring.

The damaged cervix

Recent research indicates that a necessary condition for fertility is a detectable amount of mucus. The lubricative nature of the mucus ensures that it quickly appears at the vaginal opening if sufficient quantities are produced by the cervix.

A damaged cervix can fail to produce mucus. This damage may follow surgery for pre-cancerous or cancerous growths of the cervix, or for cervical erosion, a condition in which the surface of the cervix is abnormal and may become infected. Treatment of the erosion may involve gentle removal of the damaged area with diathermy (heat), cryosurgery (cold), or sometimes with laser beams.

In the case of removals of early-stage cancers, the cervix returns to near-normal and most women can have children after such treatment. If the procedure is extensive, it may completely remove the mucus-producing area, making conception impossible.

A relatively gentle method of treatment of the cervical erosion involves repeated application of silver nitrate. This procedure allows healing of the cervix with minimal damage, so that the mucus essential for sperm vitality and transport, and for recognition of fertility, is still produced.

Production by the cervix of infertile-type mucus

If the cervix produces only infertile-type mucus this may be due to the progestogen component of contraceptive medication (p. 142), an effect which disappears spontaneously months or years after discontinuing use of oral or injected contraceptives.

Attempts have been made to stimulate production of fertile-type mucus with small doses of the chemical, Ethynyl oestradiol.

Although this results in mucus with a fertile appearance and sensation, success in achieving pregnancies has not followed. This may be due to the action of Ethynyl oestradiol in suppressing ovulation, except in very small doses.

Endometriosis

Endometriosis is the growth of endometrial tissue on the tubes, ovaries, urinary, or intestinal organs. The symptoms vary; but women troubled by painful menstrual cramps or uncomfortable intercourse and unusually long menstrual bleeding should seek medical advice.

A woman who is familiar with her normal mucus pattern may detect this abnormality at an early stage by the disturbed pattern as well as by prolonged bleeding and spotting.

If endometriosis is identified as the cause of infertility, treatment in the form of surgery or hormonal therapy may help. The surgical treatment is long and meticulous. The recent introduction of a synthetic hormone (Danazol) has been a significant contribution to the treatment of this condition.

Doctors may advise women in whom the condition is not yet well advanced to have their families as soon as possible, because of the possibility that the abnormal growth will irreversibly block the Fallopian tubes. Hormonal treatment may contribute further to the infertility. In some cases, pregnancy itself has a beneficial effect on halting the endometriosis.

Male infertility

It is important to emphasize the distinction between fertility and the other major male characteristic of virility or potency. The majority of men who are infertile are normally virile.

Much remains to be learnt about the causes and treatment of male infertility.

Known causes of male infertility include genetic factors; birth abnormalities; obstruction of the vas (the tube that carries the sperm from the testes to the penis); infections such as mumps after puberty, tuberculosis and venereal disease; chronic ill-health; and varicocele (an abnormality of the blood vessels of the testes). Rarely, the infertility results from a hormonal disturbance.

Acute feverish illnesses, emotional shock, and very frequent intercourse can also lower the sperm-count temporarily and this is one reason why too much attention should not be paid to a single sperm-count which is in the sub-fertile range.

Any investigation of infertility in men should include:

• A full medical history and physical examination.
• A Huhner's test. This enables the quality of the semen to be assessed, and a sperm count to be made, and indicates how the sperm cells are inter-acting with the fertile-type mucus.
• An assessment of psychological factors which may contribute to infertility, such as undue stress or fatigue.

The Huhner's test is a more accurate guide to sperm health than a sperm count alone. For a sperm count gives no indication of whether the sperm are able to survive in the female genital tract or of whether the technique of intercourse is effective.

Also, the 'normal range' of sperm in a whole ejaculate is 40 to 900 million. However, these counts are obtained from a masturbatory specimen which may vary greatly depending on anxiety, general health, or frequency of intercourse.

The criteria for 'normal' sperm counts have sometimes been set far too high, and in some cases, men told they are infertile on the basis of a sperm count later become fathers. A man should never be told he is infertile unless he is producing no sperm at all.

The relationship between infertility and sperm antibodies is not yet clear. However, even in women who produce these antibodies to their partner's sperm, pregnancy sometimes occurs.

Treatment of male infertility is often unsatisfactory because in more than half of the cases, no cause can be found. Even where a cause is identified, treatment is often very limited or ineffective.

Artificial insemination

Disease or injury may result in absence of sperm or gross disorders of sperm production, or may make sexual intercourse impossible even though production of healthy sperm continues normally.

The options for couples are to accept infertility, to adopt a child, or to proceed to artificial insemination. The technique is successful only if healthy sperm are introduced into fertile-type mucus; this provides confirmatory evidence of the essential nature of fertile mucus.

Artificial insemination from a donor other than the husband, introduces important ethical, medical, psychological and legal considerations.

In vitro fertilization ('Test-tube babies')

If your Fallopian tubes are damaged, but you are ovulating normally, a 'by-pass conception procedure' may be suggested.

Your husband's sperm fertilizes – in a test tube – the egg collected from your ovary during ovulation. Great care is needed to prevent infection from disrupting the process. This necessitates the use of antibiotics, which themselves are hazardous to new life.

If fertilization takes place, the developing egg can be transferred to the uterus when it is judged to be in a receptive phase.

This procedure is at a preliminary stage of development because of the complex chemistry involved and the difficulty in achieving precise timing. While the possibility of test-tube fertilization may offer hope to many infertile couples, this procedure also raises philosophical, psychological and social questions which are still to be answered.

Facing infertility

After all the investigations, a couple's chances of conception may seem to be very slight. This realization is difficult to accept and may prove extremely disheartening. If partners can think of this as something to face together, they may find that instead of separating them, it brings them closer to each other. Hardships do not cause a relationship to break down if partners can turn to each other in love.

They can fulfil their creativity in many ways. If they look around they will very likely see that many children need them.

It sometimes happens that when partners have become resigned to childlessness and have developed a contentment with each other, a pregnancy unexpectedly occurs, confounding the cleverest doctors.

13

The technological approach to contraception

While the Pill has been responsible for enabling many women to take effective control of their fertility, it has not been without its cost. In recent years, a trend away from the contraceptive Pill has become apparent. The enthusiasm of the early 1960s has been tempered by increasing caution due to reports of complications of both short- and long-term use.

This is particularly so in women over the age of thirty-five who are now advised by health authorities to find an alternative method of fertility control.

There is a trend towards sterilization and abortion; but many women find these methods unsatisfactory or unacceptable.

The ideal in fertility control should be a reliable, harmless, immediately reversible, and inexpensive method. It should not detract from the pleasure of sexual intercourse and it should encourage a good emotional and sexual relationship between partners. How do the available artificial contraceptives measure up against these criteria?

Despite the large input of money and research into new methods in recent years, most methods fall down somewhere along the line. Indeed, couples seeking to limit or space their families face a real dilemma.

Should they try alternating physical barrier methods – such as condoms or diaphragms – with the Pill or with natural methods? Should they rely on the Pill or the IUD and risk suffering their side-effects? Or does the finality of sterilization hold the only solution?

All in all, it adds up to an unappealing picture of drugs,

devices and surgical sterilization. For each couple, it is a serious and individual decision. One of the most vital considerations is the effectiveness of the various methods.

In practice, every known method of fertility control has a failure rate, and these are discussed in this and the next chapter. Some methods have a significantly lower failure rate than others – for example the IUD is less prone to failure than, say, contraceptive foam.

Yet there is a growing realization that the method failure rate is not the only consideration. What are the side-effects? Are there aesthetic objections? To what extent does success with a method depend on motivation?

It is the balancing of such factors that will finally help couples decide on a fertility control method that suits them.

Approaches to fertility control

To date the approaches to fertility control have included:
• Natural methods, where couples avoid intercourse during the fertile phase of the menstrual cycle and thus do not alter the body's natural processes. These methods are described in the next chapter.
• Sterilizing methods, where the Fallopian tubes or vas deferens are divided, or the uterus is removed, or in the case of types of Pill, where egg production is prevented.
• Contraceptive methods, where a physical or chemical barrier is placed between the sperm and the egg (e.g. with a diaphragm or condom, or a spermicidal cream), or where cervical mucus is rendered impenetrable.
• Abortive methods, where the fertilized egg cell is prevented from continuing its normal development.

In this chapter, let us examine the safety and effectiveness of various artificial methods of fertility control.

Oral Contraceptive Pill

REGULAR This is the most common type and is usually simply referred to as the Pill. It is a combination of two synthetic hormones, oestrogen and progestogen. Progestogen is a substance similar to the hormone, progesterone, which is normally produced by the ovaries.

The amount of oestrogen and progestogen varies in the thirty or so brands of the Pill now available.

In recent years, governments have legislated to reduce the hormone levels in the Pills generally available.

Effectiveness, if the Pill is taken as directed, is estimated at about 99.5 per cent.

LOW DOSE   Similar to the regular Pill, but containing lower doses of one or both of the component hormones, this may be slightly less effective than the regular Pill.

MINI PILL   A single hormone Pill, containing only a progestogen, it must be taken every day at about the same time – or within at most three hours of the usual time – to be effective (compared with an allowable twelve-hour variation in the time of taking the regular Pill). Thus you are more likely to become pregnant than if you forget to take a regular Pill. The effectiveness is estimated at about 97 per cent. The Mini Pill is often given to women who are breastfeeding.

How does the Pill work?

The regular Pill acts in a number of ways simultaneously.

First it inhibits ovulation. The hormones in the Pill replace the normal production of oestrogen and progesterone by the ovaries. They suppress the triggering mechanism in the brain which causes the release of Follicle Stimulating Hormone (FSH) and Luteinizing Hormone (LH), and thus prevent ovulation in about 98 per cent of cycles.

Secondly, the progestogen component of the regular Pill stimulates the production of barrier (infertile-type) mucus. The aim here is to prevent sperm penetration and survival, acting thus as a contraceptive.

Thirdly, the Pill disrupts the normal growth pattern of the endometrium so that it is not capable of nurturing the egg even if it is released and fertilized.

In Pills with a low dose of oestrogen (for example, 30 micrograms), the effects on sperm penetration of the mucus and on the endometrium (causing failure to implant) assume greater importance. Some studies indicate that the low dose Pills prevent ovulation only 50 per cent of the time.

The Mini Pill, containing only a progestogen, suppresses ovulation in only 40 per cent of cycles, and relies for its contraceptive effectiveness on stimulating the production of barrier-type mucus, as well as altering the normal growth of the endometrium so that it cannot support a fertilized egg. It may also alter the normal contractions of the Fallopian tubes and the function of the corpus luteum.

Effectiveness of the Pill

The variation in the effectiveness of the different forms of the Pill is due mainly to the amount of oestrogen present. When the oestrogen content is fifty micrograms or more, the Pill's estimated effectiveness in preventing pregnancy is 99.5 per cent.[1] Pills containing 20 to 35 micrograms of oestrogen have a method effectiveness of about 97 per cent.

In practice, many women forget to take the Pill occasionally, resulting in a total pregnancy rate of about seven per hundred women years. That is, among one hundred women using the Pill for a year, seven would become pregnant.[2]

Oral contraceptives must be taken every day to be effective because the oestrogen component is broken down by the body in twenty-four hours. If more than one Pill is missed, it is likely that there will be a surge of Luteinizing Hormone (LH) which will lead to the release of an egg cell later in the cycle.

Acceptability

It is important to remember that the quoted effectiveness rates apply only to the group of women who are able to tolerate the Pill. Many women cannot use oral contraceptives either because of pre-existing medical conditions or because of side-effects.

Many of the adverse side effects on health are related to the dosage of oestrogen – the higher the oestrogen content, the more likely are severe effects. However, progestogens may also cause problems.

It is because of these side-effects that many women discontinue the Pill. For example, a study of Australian women found a discontinuation rate of 51 per cent at one year.[3]

And according to Sir Richard Doll, a British authority on health statistics, of one hundred women on oral contraceptives: at the end of one year, seventy could be expected to be using the Pill; four to have switched to an IUD; two to the diaphragm; six could be expected to be pregnant; and eighteen to have given up using any form of contraception.[4]

According to Professor Harvey Carey from the University of New South Wales, as many as 33 per cent of oral contraceptive users discontinue for reasons other than desiring a pregnancy.[5] The main reasons include weight gain, headaches, decreased libido and depression, with some women reporting multiple side-effects.

When is the Pill advised against?

The US Food and Drug Administration (FDA) advises women with the following conditions not to use the Pill:[6]
- clots in the legs or lungs
- angina pectoris (pains in the heart)
- known or suspected cancer of the breast or sex organs
- unusual vaginal bleeding that has not yet been diagnosed
- known or suspected pregnancy.

Furthermore, the FDA advises any woman who in the past has suffered a heart attack or stroke, or clots in the legs or lungs, to avoid using the Pill. Conditions that your doctor will want to watch closely if you are using the Pill, or which might suggest use of an alternative method include:
- a family history of breast cancer
- breast nodules, fibrocystic disease of the breast, or an abnormal mammogram
- diabetes

- high blood pressure
- high cholesterol
- cigarette smoking
- migraine headaches
- heart or kidney disease
- epilepsy
- fibroid tumours of the uterus
- gallbladder disease
- depression.

Smokers take a substantial risk by using the Pill. According to the FDA:

> Cigarette smoking increases the risk of serious adverse effects on the heart and blood vessels from oral contraceptives use.
>
> This risk increases with age and with heavy smoking (fifteen or more cigarettes a day) and is quite marked in women over thirty-five years of age.
>
> Women who use oral contraceptives should not smoke. They are about five times more likely to have a heart attack than Pill-users who do not smoke, and about ten times more likely to have a heart attack than non-users who do not smoke.

Adverse effects of the Pill

The Pill indisputably does what it claims to do – it prevents pregnancy. But as well as fulfilling its professed function, the Pill can do many other things – some of them very unpleasant – to your body.

The most disconcerting aspect of the Pill is that it can affect virtually every organ system in the body. More than thirty known side-effects have been documented in medical journals, government health information bulletins, and advice from leading medical organizations (such as the World Health Organization, the Royal College of General Practitioners in Britain, and the US Food and Drug Administration).

Detailed warnings of possible side-effects – running to two foolscap pages – are now compulsory with Pill prescriptions in the USA. It is advisable, even crucial, to take account of these warnings.

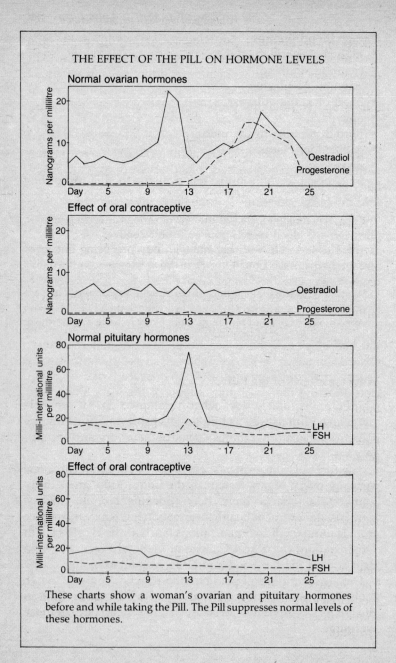

THE EFFECT OF THE PILL ON HORMONE LEVELS

Normal ovarian hormones

Nanograms per millilitre

Oestradiol
Progesterone

Day 5 9 13 17 21 25

Effect of oral contraceptive

Nanograms per millilitre

Oestradiol
Progesterone

Day 5 9 13 17 21 25

Normal pituitary hormones

Milli-international units per millilitre

LH
FSH

Day 5 9 13 17 21 25

Effect of oral contraceptive

Milli-international units per millilitre

LH
FSH

Day 5 9 13 17 21 25

These charts show a woman's ovarian and pituitary hormones before and while taking the Pill. The Pill suppresses normal levels of these hormones.

Data on the long-term consequences of the Pill are only now becoming available. The Pill has been used widely for less than twenty years, and few women have individually experienced prolonged use of it. Nor has there been the intensive medical follow-up required for proper evaluation of its long-term effects.[7]

It is known that many of the short-term complications that occur during, or shortly after, starting the Pill are associated with the heart, blood vessels, blood pressure, or changes in body chemistry.[8]

Many of the side-effects of the Pill are experienced so commonly, or are so serious, that it is worth listing some of them.

THROMBOSIS One of the most serious problems encountered when taking the Pill is that the oestrogen component tends to increase the formation of blood clots (thrombosis).[9]

Progestogen may also be involved in blood clotting, particularly in the presence of stress.[10]

The problem first became apparent in the late 1960s, after the Pill had been in general use for eight years. At that time, Oxford University researchers showed an association between use of oral contraceptives and an increased risk of blood clots affecting the veins and arteries of the legs, lungs, and brain.

It is now estimated that Pill-users are between four and eight times more likely to die of thrombosis, particularly in the presence of stress.[11]

Since 1970, on the advice of the British Committee on the Safety of Drugs, the oestrogen content has been reduced in newer formulations to no more than 30 micrograms, thus reducing the risk of thrombosis.[12] The progestogen level has also been reduced.

The formation of clots can be a serious problem when emergency surgery is required on a woman who is taking the Pill. Because of the effects on clotting, surgeons now recommend that a woman undergoing elective (non-urgent) surgery should discontinue the Pill four to eight weeks before her operation.

HEART ATTACKS   The clear identification of a relationship between heart attacks and Pill-use came in the late 1960s.

The estimated risk of a heart attack is 2.8 times higher in Pill-users than non-users.[13]

Other factors which increase this risk are high blood pressure, smoking more than fifteen cigarettes a day, high blood fat levels, and diabetes.

It is estimated that the combined effect of the Pill and two or more of these other risk factors is a disturbing 128-fold increase in the risk of a heart attack.[14] The length of use appears to be an important consideration, and even ex-users seem to be more at risk from heart attack than never-users.

Overall, the data suggest an increased annual risk of one death for every 5000 women who have at some time used the Pill; the risk is concentrated in older women, particularly those with a long duration of Pill-use and who also smoke.

HIGH BLOOD PRESSURE   An estimated 5 per cent of Pill-users will develop a mild to severe increase in blood pressure.[15] Oestrogen appears to cause this effect, by altering the lining of blood vessels. In general, older and more obese users of the Pill are more likely to develop high blood pressure. Since elevated blood pressure is a known risk factor in heart disease among Pill-users, doctors often suggest an alternative method of fertility control.

STROKE   The risk of developing a stroke is estimated to be 9.5 times greater in Pill-users than non-users.[16]

The risk increases with age and duration of Pill usage, but even in the fifteen to thirty-four year age group, the estimated excess annual death rate is comparable to road traffic accident deaths for women of the same age.[17]

In a young woman, the stroke may not be fatal, but it can have a devastating impact on the patient and her family because of the lengthy rehabilitation necessary and residual physical or mental impairment.

GALLBLADDER DISEASE   The Boston Collaborative Drug Surveillance Program has demonstrated a relationship between Pill-use and the development of gallbladder disease.[18] This relationship seems to hold for all age groups, and appears to be an effect of oestrogen. American and British studies indicate that the incidence of surgically proven gall stones is doubled in women on the Pill.[19]

LIVER TUMOURS   In recent years, several controlled studies have confirmed the relationship between Pill-use and the development of a potentially dangerous tumour of the liver. Although the tumour does not usually spread beyond the liver, the danger arises if it ruptures and bleeds excessively.

According to a 1977 report from the Center for Disease Control in Atlanta, Georgia,[20] approximately five hundred cases of this rare tumour have now been documented, although not all in Pill-users. Some of the cases have been fatal.

Typically, the tumour becomes apparent when an unexplained liver enlargement and upper abdominal pain occur in a woman who has used the Pill for seven years or more.

It is estimated that the risk of developing a liver tumour is five times more common in women who have used the Pill for five to seven years, and twenty-five times more common in those taking the Pill for nine years or more, than in women who have never taken it.[21]

BIRTH DEFECTS   US Food and Drug Administration advises women who suspect they are pregnant not to take oral contraceptives because of possible damage to the developing child.[22]

An increased risk of birth defects, including heart and limb defects, has been associated with the use of sex hormones, including oral contraceptives, in pregnancy.

In addition, the developing female child whose mother has received DES (diethylstilbestrol), an oestrogen (formerly used to prevent early miscarriage) during pregnancy has a risk of getting cancer of the vagina or cervix in her teens or young adulthood. The risk is estimated to be about one in 1000 exposures or less.

Abnormalities of the urinary and sex organs have been reported in male offspring so exposed. It is possible that other oestrogens, such as the oestrogens in oral contraceptives, could have the same effect in the child if the mother takes them during pregnancy.

Health authorities now advise women who wish to become pregnant to use another method of fertility control for three or four months after coming off the Pill before attempting to conceive. This is because of the increased incidence of foetal abnormalities found in miscarried babies whose mothers used the Pill immediately before becoming pregnant. If you do become pregnant soon after stopping use of oral contraceptives – and if you do not miscarry – there is no evidence that the baby has an increased risk of abnormality. The greatest risk lies in those cases where low dose Pills are used after an unsuspected pregnancy has occurred.

BREAST MILK QUALITY AND QUANTITY   According to the World Health Organization, there is evidence that the Pill reduces the amount of breast milk available to the baby.[23]

The quality of the milk protein may also be adversely affected.

Some national authorities have advised women either not to use the Pill while breastfeeding, or only to use it once lactation is well established.

For example, the Australian Health Department does not recommend that nursing mothers use the Mini Pill. For this has been shown to interfere with the protein content of breast milk, as well as altering the amount of calcium, sodium, potassium, phosphorus, magnesium, and fats.[24]

The hormones contained in the Pill have been shown to enter breast milk, and thus they may be absorbed by the breast-fed baby.[25] Synthetic progesterone is known to act on the hypothalamus – an important brain centre. What effect this has on the developing infant is not yet established.

It is neither wise nor advisable to prescribe oral contraceptives to nursing mothers [our italics]. This is because the steroid components (hormones), as is the case with most drugs, are excreted into the milk. Their effects on the neonate are variable and dose-dependent. For example, an androgen-type progestogen may masculinize a female infant, and steroid metabolites may contribute to neonatal jaundice.

– Dr W. N. Spellacy, Chairman, Department of Obstetrics and Gynecology, University of Miami Medical School

ECTOPIC PREGNANCY Transport in the tubes is normally under the control of both oestrogen and progesterone. Synthetic hormones disturb this mechanism. The Mini Pill is associated with a significantly increased risk of ectopic pregnancy (a pregnancy in a Fallopian tube, instead of the uterus).[26]

CANCER OF THE REPRODUCTIVE ORGANS Some types of Pill have been taken off the market because of a possible link with cancer of the endometrium, particularly with prolonged Pill-use.

The Pill also has an effect on the cervix, and may promote the progression to cancer of already abnormal cells.[27] Serious cervical erosion (p. 135), requiring treatment, is also associated with Pill-use.

BREAST TUMOURS Many studies indicate that women on the Pill have a *reduced* risk of getting benign (non-cancerous) breast disease such as breast cysts. And several studies have found no increase in breast cancer in women who already have benign breast disease. However, the US Food and Drug Administration urges watchfulness where there is a history of breast disease.[28]

Women with a strong family history of breast cancer or who have breast nodules, fibrocystic disease, or abnormal mammograms, or who were exposed to DES during their mother's pregnancy, must be followed very closely by their doctors if they choose to use oral contraceptives instead of another method of contraception.

MENSTRUAL IRREGULARITIES Breakthrough bleeding between periods commonly occurs with the low dose Pill containing 30 micrograms or less of oestrogen. This may settle down within the first few months of use. The Mini Pill (progestogen only) tends to cause continued spotting, unpredictable bleeding, or periods may stop altogether in a small number of users. Approximately 25 per cent of women prescribed the Mini Pill give it up because of unacceptable bleeding.[29]

POST-PILL INFERTILITY   This can be recognized by failure to menstruate or ovulate, or disturbance of production of the fertile-type mucus.

Post-pill amenorrhoea is the failure to menstruate within six months of coming off the Pill.

In a typical study finding, Evrard and his colleagues reported that 30 per cent of women coming off the Pill menstruated within thirty days, a further 60 per cent menstruated within sixty days, and 2 per cent had not menstruated after six months.[30]

The US Food and Drug Administration advises women with irregular menstrual cycles not to use the Pill, warning that they may have difficulty in becoming pregnant later.[31]

In some studies, more than 50 per cent of the women who developed post-Pill amenorrhoea had considerable menstrual irregularity before taking the Pill.[32] Young women of unproven fertility and light-weight women appear to be at increased risk of serious disturbance of their menstrual cycles after coming off the Pill.

A recent editorial in the *British Medical Journal* stated:[33]

Post pill amenorrhoea does not threaten health and is seldom permanent unless it is incidental to other causes of secondary amenorrhoea.

Judged by the yardstick of successful pregnancy the outlook is less rosy. Although upwards of 80 per cent of women with post pill amenorrhoea will ovulate with treatment, in a recent study only twenty-two births were obtained among fifty treated cases.

It appears that following prolonged exposure to oral contraceptives, a large proportion of mucus of the infertile type is released, or insufficient fertile-type mucus is produced. Since the lubricative fertile-type mucus is essential for sperm fertilizing capacity and transport, conception fails even though ovulation may be occurring. As yet no remedy has been found for this disturbance.

VITAMIN AND MINERAL STATUS   About one-third of women on the Pill show reduced blood levels of vitamin C, as well as being deficient in certain B group vitamins, including vitamin B12 which is needed to prevent anaemia. Reduced levels of folic acid (necessary for proper functioning of the red blood cells) also occur in about one-third of Pill-users.[34]

Diet may overcome these deficiencies once they are identified; but where diets are inadequate or unbalanced or where the vitamin deficiency is not identified, the result may be fatigue and lowered resistance to infection.

The World Health Organization is studying the vitamin status of Pill-users in various parts of the world, and looking at the potential of vitamin supplements to offset the vitamin depletion. Multi-vitamin capsules containing vitamin B6, folic acid, vitamin C, and vitamin B12 are now recommended for women taking the Pill.

Levels of trace elements which play an essential role in many chemical processes within the body are also altered by Pill use.

INFECTIONS By changing the normal environment of the reproductive tract, the Pill may encourage the growth of organisms which cause thrush and gonorrhoea. Monilial vaginitis is often troublesome and recurrent in women taking the Pill: this is due to progestogens disturbing the normal growth of the cells lining the vagina.[35]

WEIGHT GAIN Oral contraceptives alter carbohydrate metabolism in 15 to 40 per cent of women on the Pill. The hormones in the Pill tend to increase appetite, facilitate fat deposition and cause fluids to be retained which may also increase weight.[36]

MIGRAINE If the Pill sets off migraines it should be discontinued. The headaches are sometimes related to withdrawal of oestrogen in the Pill-free week of the cycle.

NAUSEA Many Pill-users complain of this especially shortly after commencing the Pill. Young women who have never been pregnant, and women who tend to experience nausea during pregnancy, seem to be worst affected.

DIABETES The insulin requirements of women on the Pill who have diabetes need to be watched carefully. Some women with preclinical diabetes that has not yet been detected, or with a family history of diabetes, may develop obvious signs of the disorder when they start using the Pill.

DEPRESSION, IRRITABILITY, LOSS OF INTEREST IN SEX   An estimated 6 per cent of women on the Pill develop irritability, loss of libido, and depression.[37] A previous history of depression appears to predispose some women to increased symptoms. The longer the time of Pill-use, the older you are, and the higher the progestogen level of the Pill, the more likely you are to suffer from these complaints.

My generation, aged thirty in 1975, has had the Pill since we were eighteen. We have had twelve years of trying it. Most of us grew up thinking 'the Pill' was synonymous with 'contraceptive'; we had no experience of any other method except abstinence. Yet I know scarcely any women who still take the Pill. All my friends and acquaintances have rejected it because they are unable to bear the depression, the weight gains, the constant feelings of irritability, the loss of sexual feeling.

The last reason figures highly in their rejection of oral contraceptives. One of the promises the Pill supposedly holds out to women is that, at last, free from worrying about whether each sexual encounter could produce a pregnancy, they will be able to relax and enjoy sex. What is offered with one hand, however, is cruelly taken away with the other.

The Pill while it protects women from the consequences of sexual relations, all too often stops them wanting any. They are afforded protection from something they no longer desire. No wonder so many women feel cheated, feel that this so-called liberator of women is just one more agent of oppression.

– Anne Summers, *Damned Whores and God's Police* (Penguin).

Overall risk

It has taken almost two decades to arrive at scientifically-based estimates of the risks to health and life, let alone possible irreversible damage to fertility, associated with the Pill.

Most of the studies on adverse effects have been conducted in Britain and the USA, and the results are summarized by the World Health Organization as follows:[38]

Non-Pill-taking British women aged 15 to 49 years have an overall death rate from cardiovascular diseases of about 5.5 per 100 000 per year.

By comparison, the death rate among Pill-users who do not smoke is estimated to be about 13.8 per 100 000 per year, and among those Pill-users who do smoke, the death rate is thought to be around 39.5 per 100 000 per year.

The risk of death increases markedly among women over the age of 35, especially if they are also smokers, are overweight, or have diabetes, and have used the Pill for a long time.

WHO says that some of the current findings apply to brands of the Pill which contain very high oestrogen doses and which are no longer in widespread use.

Restricting the analysis of the Pill's adverse effects to counting deaths, hospital admissions, and medical complications is inadequate. This approach takes no account of the personal burden so many women take upon themselves by using the Pill. Who can measure the toll on a mother of several young children who constantly suffers from Pill-associated headache, nausea, depression, irregular bleeding and loss of sexual interest?

The Intra-Uterine Device (IUD), coil, loop

IUDs come in two main types. Both work by causing an inflammatory reaction of the endometrium so that a fertilized egg cannot implant.

INERT DEVICES   These devices are considered more suitable for women who have given birth (for example the Lippes Loop).

BIOACTIVE DEVICES   These contain either copper or a synthetic progestogen, and need to be replaced every one to three years (e.g. Copper 7, Copper T, Progestasert).

After a few years, the IUD tends to lose its effectiveness, and so replacement is recommended. Studies on IUDs containing copper show that part of their effect is in reducing sperm survival. However after two years they tend to become coated with a layer of calcium, and a new device must be inserted.

Effectiveness

The method effectiveness of IUDs is estimated at between 94 and 99 per cent.[39]

This figure does not take into account those women who are advised against using an IUD (for example, because of pelvic infection, abnormal uterine bleeding, or valvular heart disease); or those in whom it is expelled; or those who have to stop using it because of adverse effects.

Side-effects of the IUD

The incidence of pregnancy, expulsion, and removal due to side-effects, is highest in the first year of use, and drops thereafter.

An IUD may be expelled from the body either soon after it is inserted, or at a later time. In four women in one hundred, the IUD will be spontaneously expelled, with a somewhat higher figure for women who have not had children, and for certain types of IUD. The device may pass from the body without a woman being aware of the fact, leaving her with the possibility of an unexpected pregnancy.

The continuation rate at one year is about 70 per cent.[40]

Some IUDs have been taken off the market because of problems discussed in the following pages. These include the M device, the Majzlin Spring, and the Dalkon Shield.

PERFORATION   Some types of IUD carry a risk of perforation of the uterus or the cervix. That is, the IUD tends to migrate into the tissues surrounding the uterus. This may result in intestinal obstruction or severe bleeding, especially if the device contains copper. At the very least, perforation results in difficulty of removal and sometimes necessitates hysterectomy, or endangers life. The device perforates the uterus in about one in 300 women using the Dalkon Shield and one in 3000 women using the Copper T.[41]

INFECTION The Dalkon Shield was withdrawn after its association with at least seventeen deaths between 1972 and 1974 was recognized in the US. It appears that the tail of the shield harboured bacteria even though the outside of the tail was sterilized.

Pelvic infections are a common and potentially dangerous problem associated with IUDs. The risk of such an infection among IUD-users is estimated to be three times higher than among non-users.[42] Women who have not had children appear to be at increased risk of infection.

Recent studies indicate that IUDs may introduce infection into the reproductive organs, or they may help invading organisms become established by their very presence.

Possible indications of an IUD-related infection are excessive, abnormal bleeding, pain or tenderness in the abdomen, severe cramps, or a persistent, profuse or offensive discharge.

If left untreated, infection can damage the delicate lining of the Fallopian tubes. The narrow channel through which the sperm and egg cell must travel may become irreparably scarred, resulting in an inoperable blockage and consequent infertility. Because of this, some doctors advise women who have not yet had their families against using an IUD.

If severe infection has damaged the uterus, a hysterectomy (removal of the uterus) may be necessary.

Treatment of an IUD-infection with antibiotics – without removing the IUD – is bad medical practice. It disregards the basic principle of treating infection caused by a foreign body – which is first to remove it.

PREGNANCY AND COMPLICATIONS As already mentioned, the IUD is between 94 and 99 per cent effective, that is up to 6 per cent of IUD-users will experience a recognized pregnancy in a year. If such a pregnancy occurs with an IUD in place, the chances of miscarriage are between 30 and 50 per cent.[43]

The device should be removed if possible when the pregnancy is confirmed. The removal may be hazardous for the child. Infection is likely to be a complicating factor.

Five to 10 per cent of pregnancies among IUD-users (i.e. three pregnancies in 1000 IUD-users) are ectopic – the fertilized egg settles in a Fallopian tube.[44] Typically, this results in a ruptured Fallopian tube about eight to twelve weeks later requiring surgical removal. Following a tubal pregnancy, conception occurs less readily and studies demonstrate a 50 to 60 per cent chance of not conceiving again at all.

A recent study for the first time reports an increase in sterility and a decrease in average ability to bear children in urban Taiwanese women using IUDs.[45] This effect appears to increase with the duration of IUD-use.

Although many pregnancies go to term with an IUD in place, there is a substantial risk of interruption to the pregnancy at any stage.

DAMAGE TO THE CERVIX   Women who have not had children often find insertion of the IUD extremely painful. This involves stretching the firm cervix with mechanical dilators.

In the process, the cervix tends to tear, and this can result in later miscarriage due to an 'incompetent cervix'. A severe shock reaction can also occur at the time of insertion.

The reason insertion is less painful for a woman with children is that under normal circumstances, the first time that the cervix is dilated is at the onset of labour. At this time various natural hormones act to soften the tissues of the cervix so that no damage is done.

MENSTRUAL DISORDERS   Women using an IUD tend to experience an increase in heavy menstrual periods, particularly in the first few months of use. This can result in anaemia. Once the IUD is removed, the bleeding usually returns to normal, if infection is not a complication.

CRAMPING AND BACKACHE   Cramping and backache are common complaints among IUD-users, particularly those who have not had children, and in whom the uterus has not previously been stretched by a pregnancy. Strong muscular contractions are experienced as the body tries to reject the foreign body.

While more and more women are turning to the IUD because of dissatisfaction with the Pill, it has not proved to be the long-term answer. Apart from the prospect of painful cramps, menstrual disorders and internal infection, some women express feelings of revulsion at having to tolerate for years at a time metal or plastic devices within their reproductive organs.

Diaphragm and spermicidal chemicals

Until the 1960s when the Pill and the IUD became popular, the diaphragm was commonly used.

When properly fitted – and this requires training by a doctor – the dome-shaped diaphragm fits over the cervix, forming a physical barrier to sperm cells.

The use of spermicidal foams, jellies, or pessaries adds a chemical barrier.

The method effectiveness is estimated at 95 per cent,[46] but this figure varies widely depending on the chemical spermicide used, proper fit and care of the diaphragm and consistent and careful use.

In practice, the total effectiveness is more like 80 per cent, due largely to incorrect positioning of the diaphragm or inadequate spermicidal foam.

The continuation rate of only 35 per cent at six months,[47] indicates that many couples find this method unsatisfactory.

Women complain that the diaphragm disrupts spontaneity, for unless she has planned ahead, she must insert the diaphragm immediately prior to intercourse. Some women routinely insert a diaphragm each evening to overcome this problem.

Some couples regard the messiness of the spermicidal foam or jelly that accompanies the diaphragm as a disadvantage.

Attempts to combine the diaphragm with the Ovulation Method have proved unsuccessful. The mucus pattern is obscured by seminal fluid and spermicidal cream, making accurate assessment of fertility or infertility difficult.

The condom, sheath, French letter

Used every time as directed, a high-quality condom is about 97 per cent effective.[48] Failure to use it carefully, so that some seminal fluid escapes either into the vagina, or even the area outside the vagina, reduces the effectiveness to about 80 per cent.[49]

The continuation rate at six months is about 56 per cent, and at one year only 22 per cent remain users.[50] This is an indication that many couples find the method either unsatisfactory or aesthetically unappealing.

Use of the condom may inhibit spontaneity, and may cause loss of an erection and consequent frustration. Sensation may be reduced because the penis is not directly touching the vagina.

The friction of an insufficiently lubricated condom can produce irritation in the vagina. Attempts to overcome this with lubricating chemicals may prove counter-productive: artificial agents introduced into the vagina tend to irritate the delicate lining cells, causing infection and sensitivity.

Coitus interruptus, withdrawal

This method has a long cultural history and involves withdrawal of the penis from the vagina just before ejaculation. The idea is to deposit the sperm outside the vagina, and well away from the tissues surrounding it. Use of the method frequently results in pregnancy because it is common for some sperm cells to be released as the penis becomes erect, well before orgasm. If sperm are deposited on the tissues round the vagina in the presence of fertile-type mucus, the sperm are able to make their way along the vagina, through the uterus, and thence to the Fallopian tubes where fertilization may occur.

The effectiveness of the withdrawal method is estimated at 70 to 80 per cent.[51] As well as its low level of effectiveness, withdrawal has a number of other disadvantages. Many couples find that they cannot relax fully because of anxiety about withdrawing in time. If used for a long time, withdrawal may lead to premature ejaculation in men. In women, it may make intercourse unsatisfactory because of failure ever to achieve orgasm.

Contraceptive injections

Depo-Provera (medroxy-progesterone) is taken in the form of an injection every three months. It prevents pregnancy by altering the normal growth of the endometrium among other modes of action. It is thought to interfere with the hypothalamus-pituitary-ovary circuit as well. The method is estimated to be 99 per cent effective. The continuation rate is about 56 per cent at one year.[52]

COMPLICATIONS Depo-Provera may cause a progressive decline in bleeding each cycle. If it continues to be used for more than two years, menstrual periods may no longer occur, probably because the endometrium is no longer capable of normal growth. Return of fertility may be delayed for months or years, or it may never return. On the other hand, the injectible contraceptive sometimes causes heavy and unpredictable bleeding.

Other problems involve the risk of congenital malformations in children if the injection fails and a pregnancy occurs. It is also known that Depo-Provera adversely affects breast milk. Headaches, depression, loss of libido and pains in the limbs are among the adverse reactions.

Some governments have restricted its availability. For example, the US Food and Drug Administration (FDA) will not approve its use for contraception in the United States because 'its benefits for this purpose to patients in the United States do not justify the risk'.[53] And the Australian Health Department and FDA have banned its use except with special permission. Nevertheless, some population agencies are still distributing it widely in developing countries.

Concern has also been expressed because cancer of the uterus has been linked with Depo-Provera in experimental animals.

Skin implants

This is a new development in which contraceptive chemicals are enclosed in a capsule and inserted under the skin. They appear to inhibit ovulation. The aim is to enclose enough contraceptive for the implant to be effective for about a year.

A recent study involving two different progestogens found that major problems were menstrual disturbances, involving irregular or prolonged bleeding or amenorrhoea; infection at the site of implantation; a slight increase in weight; headaches and acne.

About one-third of women discontinued use of the implant during the first year.

Sterilization

Sterilization is a fundamental life change and is therefore an extremely difficult and serious step.

With present surgical techniques, reversal attempts are rarely successful. This can prove a source of great regret should the family situation change – through death of a child or re-marriage – and another child be desired. It should be regarded as irreversible.

Female sterilization procedures

HYSTERECTOMY   This involves removal of the uterus, and usually the cervix also. The woman continues to ovulate, but menstruation, fertilization and implantation no longer happen.

TUBAL LIGATION   There are two ways of doing this, both requiring a local or general anaesthetic. In one, a fairly large abdominal incision is made, a piece of each Fallopian tube is cut out, and the two ends are tied off and folded back into the surrounding tissue. This method is often used immediately after childbirth. The second method involves entering the body through the vagina and cutting the tubes. After these procedures, menstruation continues as the uterus is still intact.

THE ENDOSCOPIC OR ELECTRO-COAGULATION TECH-
NIQUE   This involves burning the tubes with a small instrument introduced into the body either through an abdominal
incision or through the vagina.

USE OF A CLIP RING TO CLOSE OFF THE FALLOPIAN
TUBE   This causes the tube to become fibrous. In a small
number of cases, this type of sterilization has been reversed
and a subsequent pregnancy achieved. However most doctors
advise that the operation is permanent.

Microsurgery is increasingly being used when reversal procedures are requested. However even the best surgeons are
unable to reverse more than 50 per cent of these operations.

It is now the policy of some hospitals not to perform steriliza-
tions within a few days of birth. For while domestically ideal,
in that the mother is not hospitalized for an extended period, it
is a time of emotional flux, during which a decision that may be
regretted later might easily be made.

EFFECTIVENESS   Not surprisingly, the method effectiveness
of either male or female sterilization is almost 100 per cent.

COMPLICATIONS OF TUBAL LIGATION   Physical complications of tubal sterilization include severe bleeding, pelvic infection, and ectopic pregnancies. The ectopic pregnancy-rate
following tubal ligation is reported to be twenty times the
normal rate. The reported incidence of menstrual problems
such as heavy bleeding varies from 8 to 25 per cent.[54] In about
one-third of women who have had a tubal ligation, the blood
supply to the uterus is disturbed due to interference with the
blood vessels of the Fallopian tubes. This may necessitate a
hysterectomy.

COMPLICATIONS OF A HYSTERECTOMY   Post-operative
depression and sexual dysfunction are more common after a
hysterectomy than after other operations.[55] Depression requiring psychiatric referral is about three times more common than
after other operations. Fears concerning a hysterectomy tend
to be deep-seated. They may centre around a possible loss of

femininity, loss of childbearing ability, and effects on sexuality.

The two major sexual problems following hysterectomy are loss of interest in sex, and dyspareunia (pain with intercourse). In a study of sexual response following hysterectomy and removal of ovaries, one-third of women complained of a deterioration of their sexual relationships, which they attributed to the operation.[56]

Pelvic infection is a complication in about one per cent of cases.

Male sterilization

The operation is called a vasectomy, and involves a local anaesthetic followed by incisions in the scrotum. The doctor locates the right and left vas deferens (the tubes through which sperm from the testes travel to the penis); a piece of each is removed, and the ends tied off.

Following vasectomy, the presence of sperm cells has been demonstrated for three weeks to three months making conception possible during this time.[57, 58, 59, 60]

Techniques to re-join the vas are being developed by microsurgeons, but even when they have been successful, normal sperm function does not always return. Doctors advise men contemplating the operation to regard it as irreversible.

COMPLICATIONS Complications of vasectomy include infection and haemorrhage. Recent research also indicates that sperm not ejaculated from the body are broken down and pass into the bloodstream. There antibodies to the retained sperm are produced. Suspected consequences include thyroid and joint disorders, heart and circulatory diseases, and diabetes.[61]

It is estimated that 10 per cent of men who have a vasectomy experience some psychological problems as a result. For instance, some men who feel they are not whole after the operation experience severe anxiety and loss of self-esteem.

From a wide number of species there is alarming evidence that vasectomy can cause widespread alterations in body chemistry of a type which might contribute to heart and circulatory diseases.

These are questions which urgently need to be followed up in human beings.

Vasectomy seems to be a very simple operation, but people have been taking too limited and short-term a view of it. The body does not like being attacked, even in simple ways surgically, and can pay you back in the most roundabout fashion.

– Dr Malcolm Carruthers, Head, Clinical Laboratory Service, Maudsley Hospital and Institute of Psychiatry, London.[62]

Conclusion

Technological attempts to find new forms of contraception continue. But at each turn, the health and well-being of a group or groups of men and women appear to be adversely affected.

The good news is that during the past decade, attention has increasingly focused on natural methods of controlling fertility. This pressure to find nature's solution has come from the community in general, as well as from scientific research teams.

The results of this reaching out towards a natural method, applicable in all circumstances of reproductive life, have proved fruitful ... as the next chapter shows.

14

Natural methods of fertility control

As dissatisfaction with contraceptive drugs and devices grows, increasing numbers of women are seeking a fertility control method that is natural – that does not interfere with the body's normal processes.

We now know that nature has provided various indications that ovulation is occurring, or has occurred. These indications have been studied, and several different methods of natural fertility control devised.

The main candidates are the Rhythm Method, the Basal Body Temperature Method, the Sympto-Thermal Method, and the Ovulation Method. How do they compare?

This chapter aims to spell out the differences between these four major categories of natural fertility control. It is important to distinguish between them because they are quite different, and much confusion surrounds them.

The success of any of these natural methods depends primarily on how well it enables you to recognize the fertile and infertile phases of your menstrual cycle.

In addition, motivation and co-operation are essential; for all natural methods require that you avoid sexual intercourse (and genital contact) when you recognize fertility.

The Rhythm Method

The Rhythm Method (also known as the Calendar Method) is based on the fact that ovulation usually takes place ten to sixteen days before the following menstrual period.

When cycles are regular, the method works well. Couples can calculate when ovulation will occur, and can avoid intercourse for some days before and after it.

The calculations are based on a study of your own cycle length over six to twelve months, taking into account the shortest and longest cycles experienced.

For example, if you record cycle lengths varying from twenty-seven to thirty-one days, you would calculate that ovulation might occur on day 11 (27 minus 16) at the earliest, or on day 21 (31 minus 10) at the latest. So abstinence would be recommended between day 11 and day 21, and for a further three to five days at the beginning (before day 11) because of possible sperm survival. This would mean, using a cycle variation of 27–31, that the early safe days would be 1–6 and the late safe days 22 until the cycle ended. If it were a twenty-seven day cycle, this would allow six days for intercourse before ovulation and six days afterwards. If it were a thirty-one day cycle, the number of late safe days would be ten.

However, as soon as any irregularity occurs – and this can happen simply as a result of emotional shock, travel, illness, after a pregnancy, or as you approach the menopause – the calculation of ovulation becomes unreliable.

Studies of the cycle length of women show that no woman is naturally regular all the time, even excluding identifiable stress situations.

The method effectiveness is 99 per cent when cycles are regular; but with irregularity it can drop to 53 per cent.[1]

The Rhythm Method is not reliable enough for most couples who wish to avoid a pregnancy. It is also unnecessarily restrictive. It has been abandoned in virtually all natural family planning programmes as a method in isolation, although it is still used combined with temperature and mucus recordings in the Sympto-Thermal method.[2]

The Basal Body Temperature Method

At the time of ovulation or shortly after, there is a small but definite elevation in your body temperature. As you remember from the chapter on the menstrual cycle, this is due to an increase in the hormone, progesterone.

The basal temperature, taken daily at the same time and under the same conditions – whenever possible after a period of rest or sleep – is at its lowest level before ovulation.

After ovulation, the temperature normally rises – a significant shift being at least 0.4°F (about 0.2°C).[3]

Advocates of the Temperature Method use different approaches when estimating the safe days for intercourse after ovulation. Some claim that a rise above a set (individually determined) temperature indicates that ovulation has occurred, while others identify this event when three temperature readings are higher than the previous six. Some advise that the temperature is taken orally, others vaginally, still others rectally.

If you are using the Temperature Method it is wise to have two thermometers and compare their readings, one with the other. This ensures continuity of an accurate record if one is broken during a critical part of the cycle.

There are several problems associated with use of the Temperature Method.

First, the temperature shift provides only a *retrospective* indication that ovulation has occurred ... so you are given no warning of ovulation and of your increasing fertility. This means that to be sure of avoiding a pregnancy you need to abstain during the first part of the cycle until the temperature rise indicates that ovulation has occurred. This may involve lengthy and unnecessary periods of abstinence particularly when cycles are long or when ovulation does not take place at all – which may be the common pattern after coming off the Pill, while breastfeeding, or when approaching the menopause.

Second, the temperature readings can be misleading. A false high temperature may follow a fever or high alcohol intake. If you were to rely on this reading as an indication that ovulation had occurred, pregnancy could result. Some studies indicate also that even when ovulation does occur, the temperature either may not rise significantly, or may do so in steps which make accurate interpretation extremely difficult.[4]

Third, the requirement that the temperature is taken at the same time of day under resting conditions may prove difficult in many family situations; such as with a mother who gets up during the night to tend young children, or when a woman is working variable shifts. For it is important to take your temperature as soon as you wake, before any activity. The term 'basal body temperature' refers to the temperature of the body at complete rest.

The effectiveness of the Temperature Method depends to a large extent on the motivation of couples and how reliably the temperature is taken under resting conditions.

Three early studies demonstrated a method effectiveness of 76 to 86 per cent (that is, of one hundred women using the temperature method for a year to avoid pregnancy, 14 to 24 would become pregnant).[5] A more recent study conducted in 1968 found a rate of effectiveness of about 93 per cent,[6] when intercourse was restricted to the days after the temperature rise.

The Temperature Method is valuable when a woman is ovulating but has some abnormality (e.g. a damaged cervix) which destroys the mucus pattern and prevents use of the Ovulation Method.

The Sympto-Thermal Method

The Sympto-Thermal Method combines certain features of the Basal Body Temperature Method and the Ovulation Method. That is, both temperature and cervical mucus are used to assess the state of fertility.

The early safe days are calculated by studying cycles over six to twelve months. These calculations and the temperature shift evaluation are modified in some of the variants by mucus observations. Other physiological indicators of fertility are taken into account, e.g. pain, breast tension, condition of the cervix, etc.

Many people find the Sympto-Thermal Method satisfactory

during normal circumstances. Most women ovulate fairly regularly for most of their reproductive life. When a woman enters a breastfeeding phase or approaches menopause, the accent of the Sympto-Thermal Method must change and Rhythm calculations and temperature readings need to give precedence to the mucus.

In managing the early days of the cycle, if precedence is given to Rhythm observations, abstinence will increase as cycles progressively lengthen due to ovulation occurring later in the cycle. When ovulation fails to occur, abstinence will be total.

The main problem with combining methods is that if different signals of ovulation are in disagreement, confusion, anxiety and abstinence tend to result, and fertility control becomes much more complicated than it need be.

Hormonal studies have shown that the mucus is the most reliable signal of fertility. If a less accurate indicator is allowed to assume prime importance, it will be difficult to transfer confidence to the mucus signals when ovulation fails and the temperature ceases to rise.

Pregnancy rates following use of the Sympto-Thermal Method vary according to the study, and the variant of the method used. A survey of Australian Natural Family Planning Centres estimated a Sympto-Thermal method-related pregnancy rate of 2.5 per cent on average, and an overall pregnancy rate of 12.3 per cent after a year of use.[7] (This figure includes pregnancies due to misunderstanding the method or choosing to disregard the guidelines.)

The Ovulation Method

As already described the basis of the method is a woman's own awareness of the mucus produced by the cervix. This provides a recognizable and scientifically validated guide to her state of fertility.

The method is applicable to all phases of reproductive life – regular cycles, irregular and anovulatory cycles, breastfeeding, approaching the menopause, and after coming off the Pill.

Other natural methods which rely on regularity of cycles are inadequate in many of these situations, and may fail at a time of great need.

Repeated studies indicate an average method-related pregnancy rate of 1 to 3 per cent (see chapter 16 describing trials of the method). This means that if one hundred couples use the method *according to the guidelines* for a year, between one and three pregnancies will result.

This rate of effectiveness compares extremely well with other fertility control methods such as the Pill and IUD (see chapter 13).

In actual use, more pregnancies may occur, due to misunderstanding of the method or inadequate teaching (0–6 per cent pregnancy rate) or a decision not to follow the guidelines, giving an overall pregnancy rate of about 20 per cent.

Most women will be able to learn the method by carefully reading this book, and, should any difficulties or uncertainty arise, seeking the assistance of an accredited Ovulation Method teacher.

There is no doubt that women do have an inbuilt set of fertility signals, and an increasing number of women are finding the use of these signals a liberating experience.

Scientific research on the Billings Method

The importance of the mucus as nature's signal of fertility has been recognized during the past twenty years. Scientific research has gradually unfolded its vital role in assisting new life to begin. Let us examine the fundamental findings of this research.

Phases of the cycle

The Ovulation Method is based on established chemical events of the menstrual cycle. The menstrual cycle can be divided into four phases:

1. *The bleeding phase or menstruation.* This is a convenient marker of the beginning and end of the cycle.
2. *The early infertile days.* These occupy a variable number of days for different women. They are prolonged for many weeks in very long cycles, and are minimal in very short cycles.
3. *The fertile phase.* During this time the cervix produces fertile mucus and the ovary releases an egg cell. This wave of fertility occupies different time spans according to the couple concerned (on average five to seven days).
4. *The late infertile days.* These begin after ovulation and the death of the egg cell. Infertility continues for the remainder of the cycle and until the cervix produces fertile mucus in the next cycle.

Ovulation and fertility

Early in the cycle the chances of a pregnancy occurring are practically nil; then if intercourse takes place about twelve hours before ovulation, up to 50 per cent of couples will achieve a pregnancy. Fertility declines rapidly to zero again in the twenty-four hours following ovulation.[1]

Not every menstrual cycle has a fertile phase. Various studies indicate that 6 to 11 per cent of cycles in healthy women are anovular (that is, no egg is released and so a pregnancy cannot occur).

Conception will occur only in ovulatory cycles, of course, and then only if intercourse occurs at an appropriate time of the cycle and if mucus of a suitable type is produced by the cervix.

Hormonal events of the cycle

The changes in the mucus reflect a highly complex chain of events in the body's hormonal system.

As the cycle begins, the pituitary gland at the base of the brain starts to produce two chemical messengers, Luteinizing Hormone (LH) and Follicle Stimulating Hormone (FSH).

The over-riding control of FSH and LH production occurs in the area of the brain called the hypothalamus.

The hypothalamus acts like a computer – analysing nerve signals from other areas of the brain, including those generated by emotions and environmental factors such as light and dark; as well as assessing hormone signals relevant to fertility.

The follicles (that is, the groups of immature eggs each contained in a sphere of cells) within the ovaries have a threshold requirement for FSH below which no stimulation occurs (that is, the FSH has to reach a certain level in the bloodstream before the follicles will start developing).

During the early infertile days of the cycle, the FSH level is below the threshold, and the mucus is commonly sparse and dense, or absent altogether. These days when no change occurs are recognized as a Basic Infertile Pattern of dryness or of mucus (chapter 4).

Once the FSH level passes the threshold, a group of follicles begins to develop. These follicles produce the hormone, oestrogen. At this point, if you have experienced dry days, you will notice mucus; if opaque, sticky mucus has been evident, you will now notice that it too, reaches a point of change.

If FSH production is arrested at this intermediate stage, the follicles remain in a state of chronic minimal stimulation which may lead to the intermittent appearance of fertile-type mucus and episodes of bleeding, indicative of some growth of the lining of the uterus, the endometrium.

Ovulation is delayed until a further rise in FSH.

This situation of delayed ovulation occurs in some cycles due to stress or illness, and is common towards the end of breastfeeding, after coming off the Pill, and when approaching the menopause.

When a follicle is developing satisfactorily, it produces the hormone oestradiol, an oestrogen, which acts as a signal informing the brain of the level of ovarian activity.

In response to a high oestradiol level, the pituitary gland slows down its production of FSH and releases a series of surges of LH over a period of forty-eight hours. The dominant follicle rapidly matures and important changes take place in the chromosomes of the egg cell – which contain the inherited genetic material.

This peak LH level triggers ovulation about seventeen hours later. The LH is also responsible for the production of the corpus luteum which forms from the empty follicle and surrounding cells in the ovary after the release of the egg.

After ovulation, the corpus luteum produces the hormones progesterone and oestradiol. These are necessary for the continued growth and development of the nutritive endometrium in preparation for possible implantation should a sperm fertilize the egg.

In the absence of pregnancy, the production of these hormones declines after about ten days, thus removing the hormonal support for the endometrium. When this is shed, menstrual bleeding occurs, and the cycle starts again with a rise of FSH.

A number of other hormones may play a role in the menstrual cycle, but their significance has yet to be established.

Development of the Billings Ovulation Method

In developing the method, four overlapping stages were involved:

• Careful clinical observation of women during many hundreds of cycles to establish a pattern of mucus recognizable by women and a set of guidelines for effective fertility control
• Scientific verification of these guidelines
• Trials to establish the effectiveness of the method
• Design of a teaching programme and training of Ovulation Method teachers.

The first breakthrough – unscrambling the mucus changes

By the mid-1960s, the mucus was thought to be a recognizable marker of fertility in about 80 per cent of women only. As a result, Rhythm calculations and temperature measurements were also taught where mucus awareness alone did not appear adequate.

However, two problems remained.

Using Rhythm calculations, seven days at most at the beginning of the cycle could be considered infertile, and thus available for intercourse. This imposed severe restrictions during breastfeeding, naturally occurring long cycles, and in the years approaching the menopause when cycles tend to be long and ovulation is an increasingly rare event. (Some attempts were made to shorten cycles artificially using hormones – an approach we rejected. We also resisted the practice of advising young mothers to stop feeding their babies so that they would ovulate.)

Couples who relied on a temperature rise to indicate post-ovulatory infertility often faced long periods of unnecessary abstinence when ovulation did not occur at all in some cycles.

The solutions to both these problems were found by paying greater attention to the mucus observations and sensations of women themselves.

It became apparent that when women taught each other the Ovulation Method, virtually all women (not 80 per cent, as the male teachers had thought) were able to produce a recognizable mucus pattern. This meant that mucus observations alone were adequate for the detection of ovulation.

It was also noticed that before the mucus began its rapid development leading to the Peak, many women were experiencing a 'positive sensation of nothingness', which they referred to as 'dry days'.

The concentrated investigation of all the 'difficult cases' – that is, breastfeeding mothers and pre-menopausal women – led to a detailed study of the long anovulatory situations. It was gradually appreciated that dryness or an unvarying scant mucus continued for a long time until a few days before ovulation, and was then replaced by mucus with the well-recognized fertile characteristics. The number of dry days or days of unchanging mucus was seen to vary according to the length of the cycle – being greater in cycles when ovulation was delayed.

It was at last appreciated that the mucus observations and sensations could tell a woman all she needed to know of the fertility both before and after ovulation. The problem of the long cycle, or the cycle in which ovulation does not occur, was thus solved.

The final refinement of the Ovulation Method occurred in 1971 when temperature recordings ceased being taught as part of the method: all attention was given to the signs of the mucus. Following this, a rapid increase in knowledge of the mucus as an indicator of fertility or gynaecological abnormalities occurred. For the first time the 'problem cases' were solved, and it remained only to verify and disseminate this information by organizing a competent teaching service.

Investigation of pregnancies

An important aspect of the clinical research has been careful investigation of all planned and unplanned pregnancies among Ovulation Method users. In particular, much attention is now directed towards trying to establish why pregnancy occurs in about 1 to 3 per cent of couples who adhere to the guidelines for avoiding a pregnancy.

Hormone studies

Much of the early key research into the method was carried out by Professor James Brown from Melbourne University and Professor Henry Burger from Monash University.

Between them they have monitored the reproductive hormones of hundreds of women using the Ovulation Method over thousands of cycles.

In 1962, Professor Brown commenced hormonal studies in Melbourne with the aim of assessing the validity of the mucus observations and sensations as indicators of fertility.

Professor Brown had earned the name Mr Oestrogens while assistant director of the Clinical Endocrinology Research Unit at Edinburgh University. His work in Edinburgh involved helping sub-fertile couples achieve a pregnancy. This was found to be possible by timing intercourse to coincide with laboratory measures of the peak level of the hormone, oestrogen.

This approach proved relatively successful, but Professor Brown later confirmed that *women's own awareness of their cervical mucus could indicate ovulation even more accurately than oestrogen measurements.*

While working in conjunction with other researchers engaged in the direct visualization of the abdominal and pelvic organs by laparoscopy, Professor Brown also helped establish the relationship between oestrogen and progesterone hormones, the cervical mucus changes, and ovulation.

He concluded that the use of the mucus as a signal of fertility or infertility, and the guidelines of the Ovulation Method, had a sound scientific basis.

While Professor Brown worked on oestrogen and progesterone hormones, Professor Burger, who now heads the Medical Research Centre at Prince Henry's Hospital in Melbourne, was engaged in pioneering work on other hormones

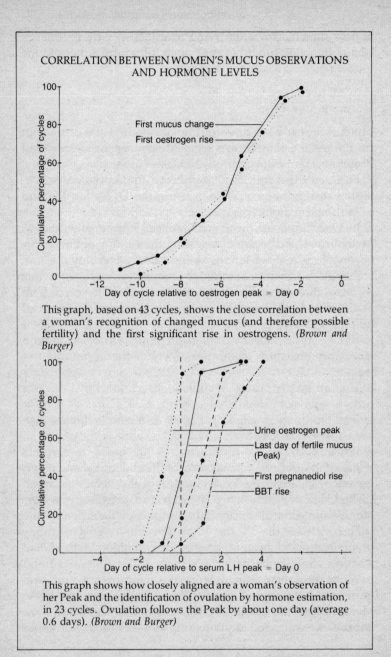

CORRELATION BETWEEN WOMEN'S MUCUS OBSERVATIONS AND HORMONE LEVELS

First mucus change

First oestrogen rise

Cumulative percentage of cycles

Day of cycle relative to oestrogen peak = Day 0

This graph, based on 43 cycles, shows the close correlation between a woman's recognition of changed mucus (and therefore possible fertility) and the first significant rise in oestrogens. *(Brown and Burger)*

Urine oestrogen peak

Last day of fertile mucus (Peak)

First pregnanediol rise

BBT rise

Cumulative percentage of cycles

Day of cycle relative to serum L H peak = Day 0

This graph shows how closely aligned are a woman's observation of her Peak and the identification of ovulation by hormone estimation, in 23 cycles. Ovulation follows the Peak by about one day (average 0.6 days). *(Brown and Burger)* which regulate the menstrual cycle. These include Follicle Stimulating Hormone (FSH) and Luteinizing Hormone (LH).

Using blood samples provided by Ovulation Method learners, Professor Burger was able to chart the changes in LH (which triggers ovulation) and FSH (which stimulates the development of the follicle containing the egg cell) during the cycles of normally fertile women. Professors Brown and Burger, working with Dr Kevin Catt, also showed that the release of LH followed the mid-cycle oestrogen peak.[2]

The first report of the work relating hormone changes to the mucus symptom was published in 1972 in *Lancet*, the British medical journal.[3] This report established the relationship between the surge of LH, ovulation, and the observation of the Peak mucus signal by a group of women.

These findings have since been confirmed by Flynn[4] in Britain, Casey[5] in Australia, Cortesi[6] in Italy and Hilgers[7] in the United States.

Further studies of these relationships have been conducted under the direction of the World Health Organization's expanded programme of research, development, and research training in human reproduction.

The available evidence indicates that:

• The oestradiol spurt resulting in fertile-type mucus that warns of possible fertility, starts on average six days before ovulation.

• The oestradiol peak occurs about thirty-seven hours before ovulation.

• The LH level begins to rise about thirty to forty hours before ovulation, reaching a peak about seventeen hours before the egg cell is released.

• The Peak mucus signal, as judged by women themselves, occurs on average 0.6 day (fourteen hours) before ovulation. In about 85 per cent of women the Peak occurs within a day of ovulation and in about 95 per cent within two days. See the diagram on page 180 which illustrates these relationships.

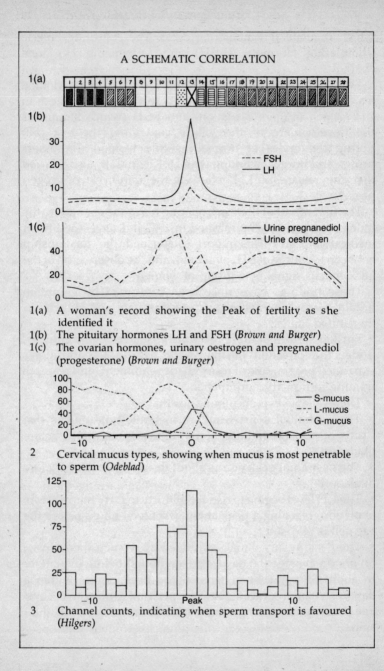

A SCHEMATIC CORRELATION

1(a)

1(b)

FSH
LH

1(c)

Urine pregnanediol
Urine oestrogen

1(a) A woman's record showing the Peak of fertility as she identified it

1(b) The pituitary hormones LH and FSH (*Brown and Burger*)

1(c) The ovarian hormones, urinary oestrogen and pregnanediol (progesterone) (*Brown and Burger*)

S-mucus
L-mucus
G-mucus

2 Cervical mucus types, showing when mucus is most penetrable to sperm (*Odeblad*)

3 Channel counts, indicating when sperm transport is favoured (*Hilgers*)

Mucus studies

Studies of the cervical mucus, particularly in relation to infertility research, have confirmed that the mucus must have special characteristics if sperm are to reach and fertilize an egg.[8]

These special characteristics give the fertile mucus its lubricativeness, and its stringy, raw egg-white appearance.

Since the late 1950s, Professor Eric Odeblad and his colleagues at the University of Umea in Sweden, have investigated the biological and physical properties of the cervical mucus.[9] They have demonstrated that three different types of mucus are produced by specialized parts of the cervix during the menstrual cycle. This mucus production is under the control of hormones, in particular, oestrogen and progesterone.

The different types of mucus either impede or encourage the movement of sperm through the reproductive system. The relative amount of each type is crucial in determining a woman's state of fertility.

The mucus during the early infertile days is composed largely of protein fibres which form an impenetrable barrier to sperm cells. This barrier mucus is characteristically opaque and sticky; and it has been termed the G-type mucus by Professor Odeblad.

The next type of mucus to appear is characterized by beads or 'loafs' of mucus, giving it a thick, clumpy texture. If stretched between the fingers, this bead-like structure is evident. Professor Odeblad has named this mucus the L-type.

When spread on a glass slide and examined microscopically, this loaf mucus shows a flower-like arrangement of perpendicularly-branched crystals.

It is a woman's awareness of this L-type mucus that signals a change from the Basic Infertile Pattern (p. 42).

At first, this L-type mucus mixes with the barrier mucus. Then, it eventually replaces it completely.

The L-type mucus has a number of very important functions: it neutralizes the acidic vagina so that sperm can survive. (Normally the vagina is inhospitable to sperm survival, and it is only in the presence of this protective mucus that sperm

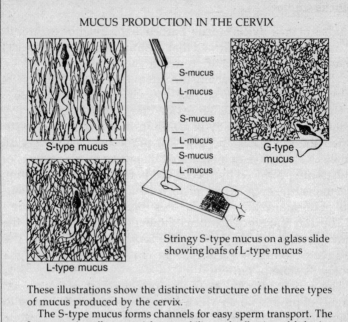

MUCUS PRODUCTION IN THE CERVIX

S-type mucus

S-mucus
L-mucus
S-mucus
L-mucus
S-mucus
L-mucus

G-type mucus

Stringy S-type mucus on a glass slide showing loafs of L-type mucus

L-type mucus

These illustrations show the distinctive structure of the three types of mucus produced by the cervix.

The S-type mucus forms channels for easy sperm transport. The L-type mucus allows partial penetrability and collection of defective sperm cells. The G-type mucus forms an impenetrable barrier.

At ovulation, S mucus predominates. After ovulation, the proportion of impenetrable G mucus increases rapidly. *(after Odeblad)*

retain their ability to fertilize an egg.) The L-type mucus also plays a part in trapping defective sperm cells. Another import-ant function is to provide a structural support for the third type of mucus, known as the S-type fertile mucus.

When the mucus can be stretched, a property of the S-type mucus, the L-type mucus is seen as beads or 'loafs' at intervals along it.

This S-type mucus indicates a high level of fertility and has a lubricative quality, resembling raw egg-white. Due to its lubricative nature, it quickly appears at the entrance to the vagina, where it produces a sensation of wetness. If stretched it forms strings or loops.

Women with normal fertility become aware of the onset of the L-type and S-type mucus on average six days before ovulation, with a range of three to ten days.[10]

Some other women may observe or feel the presence of the fertile-type mucus for only half a day, and in some cycles only.

Research on infertile couples shows that the presence of this S-type mucus, which produces a characteristic ferning pattern when spread on a glass slide, is essential if conception is to occur.[11]

On microscopic examination, the ferning pattern is seen to be due to the presence of *channels* within the S-type mucus.

Professor Thomas Hilgers from Creighton University in Omaha, Nebraska, has examined the precise nature of these channels and their part in assisting the rapid transport of sperm to the Fallopian tubes.[12]

He has found that as fertility increases during the fertile phase of the cycle, so too do the number of channels.

These channels, which form within the S-type mucus, are supported by the L-type mucus.

Professor Hilgers has studied the relationship between the channel count of the mucus taken from the cervix and women's assessment of their state of fertility or infertility based on their mucus observations and sensations.[13]

These investigations have relied upon a special technique to obtain and assess the mucus. The technique involves removing a sample of mucus from the middle of the cervical canal, preparing it for examination on a microscope slide, and then examining it under magnification. The women involved in these studies made no internal examinations themselves.

Professor Hilgers has found a very close statistical correlation between the women's assessments of their state of fertility, and the channel data.

At the time of ovulation, about 400 of these channels are typically present in the area of the cervix and the vagina. The channel number is greater on the day of the Peak, as determined by women themselves.

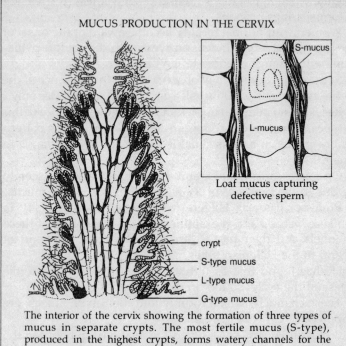

MUCUS PRODUCTION IN THE CERVIX

S-mucus

L-mucus

Loaf mucus capturing
defective sperm

crypt

S-type mucus

L-type mucus

G-type mucus

The interior of the cervix showing the formation of three types of mucus in separate crypts. The most fertile mucus (S-type), produced in the highest crypts, forms watery channels for the transport of sperm. This type of mucus occurs closest to the Peak.

The loaf mucus (L-type) eliminates defective sperm and provides a scaffolding to support the fertile (S-type) mucus.

The impenetrable (G-type) mucus is formed in the lowest crypts. *(after Odeblad)*

Professor Hilgers confirmed that these channels within the fertile-type mucus enable the cervix to act as a type of gate or biological valve, providing a passage along which the sperm cells move to the Fallopian tubes where conception takes place.

Professor Odeblad has provided supporting evidence that these channels act as a passageway at about the time of the Peak, and that their absence after the Peak removes the possibility of sperm entry. He has also shown that sperm may proceed directly to the uterus and Fallopian tubes, or may remain for a time in the specialized folds within the cervix where the S-type mucus is produced. These 'resting' sperm cells appear to be reactivated on contact with fluid from the uterus. *This mechanism of rest and reactivation explains how the life of sperm may be prolonged for several days after a single act of intercourse.*

Once the sperm cells reach the uterus and Fallopian tubes they do not live for long.

Professor Odeblad has found that the fertile S-type mucus usually *begins* to be replaced by the barrier G-type mucus just prior to ovulation.

However, some channels persist for a day after ovulation, making possible the fertilization of an egg cell for its entire lifespan, which is about twelve hours.[14]

The infertile G-type mucus gradually obscures and then replaces the fertile-type mucus.

Professor Hilgers and others have demonstrated an increased water content of the mucus at ovulation.[15, 16] This ensures its prompt arrival at the vaginal opening, eliminating the need for a woman to examine her own cervix.

The validity of mucus observations and sensations

The research has provided indisputable evidence that the hormonal and mucus events of the cycle correlate extremely well with a woman's observations and sensations. The close correlation is illustrated on p. 180.

Since even small amounts of fertile mucus produced by the cervix can be seen or felt at the vaginal opening, a woman's mucus awareness provides an effective and reliable guide to the early and late infertile days, as well as the fertile time around the Peak.

Nature has indeed provided a marker of fertility.

Scientists from many countries have confirmed the validity of the mucus observations and sensations, and in so doing have clarified the complex interplay of events involved in fertility.

Trials of the method

The variety of methods and terms used in clinical trials makes evaluation and comparison of fertility control methods extremely difficult. This chapter aims to clear a path through the jungle of words so that you can form judgements about the effectiveness, reliability, and acceptability of the Ovulation Method relative to other methods. First, an explanation of some of the terms used frequently in trials.

Trials terminology

THE METHOD-RELATED PREGNANCY RATE   This indicates the number of pregnancies, expressed as a percentage, occurring when couples carry out correct instructions for a particular method. The correctly assessed pregnancy rate under these circumstances is an indication that the method has not covered a percentage of biological circumstances.

All fertility control methods have such failures, including the Pill, the IUD and even sterilization (chapter 13). The reasons for these failures are generally unknown.

Trials indicate that the method-related pregnancy rate for the Ovulation Method is 0.5 to 2.9 per cent. This means that of 100 women using the method for a year *who consistently follow the guidelines*, between one and three may become pregnant.

THE TEACHING-RELATED PREGNANCY RATE   This figure applies to pregnancies resulting from incorrect teaching of a method, or to misunderstanding by the user of the method.

The user carries out the instructions as she or he understands them, but the misunderstanding is apparent to an experienced teacher or doctor.

With regard to the Ovulation Method, this figure varies between 0 and 6 per cent.

The variation depends largely on the calibre of the teaching. Where the teacher is committed to the success of the method and is competent and experienced, the teaching-related failure rate has been reduced to zero.

CONTINUATION RATE   This is a guide to the acceptability of a method and is judged by the readiness of users to continue with a method over an extended period and to return to a particular method after a pregnancy. The willingness to continue with the method after a pregnancy indicates that the circumstances of the pregnancy were understood and were under the control of the couple.

Because their fertility is intact, both the options to avoid or achieve a pregnancy are open to users, and they may decide to change their options from time to time.

Generally, where teaching is good, the trials of the Ovulation Method show a high continuation rate (see p. 72).

THE TOTAL PREGNANCY RATE   This total figure includes pregnancies resulting from a failure of a particular method to cover all biological circumstances, misunderstanding of the method, risk-taking by couples, ambivalence towards pregnancy, and the decision by a couple to exercise the second option of achieving a pregnancy.

Within the total pregnancy rate there may also be a number of pregnancies resulting from an act of intercourse when agreement fails between partners.

In any trial of any fertility control method a participating couple may choose to ignore the guidelines.

Personal or family reasons may lead a couple to opt out of a trial by ignoring the instructions for effective use of the particular method under study. This is the right of all couples: without this guiding principle, individual needs are displaced.

The total pregnancy rate in trials of the Ovulation Method varies between about 14 per cent and 25 per cent. This is to say that about between 14 and 25 pregnancies occur among one hundred couples participating in an Ovulation Method trial for a year.

The Ovulation Method allows both the option to avoid as well as to achieve a pregnancy and thus the total pregnancy rate is relatively high, and varies considerably from trial to trial. Some other fertility control methods do not allow couples the second option to the same degree and therefore it is to be expected that the *total* pregnancy rate relating to them will be smaller.

THE PEARL INDEX Most of the pregnancy rates quoted for the Pill, IUD, condom, and other fertility control methods are Pearl Index figures. These refer to the various types of pregnancy rate and indicate the number of pregnancies occurring for each '100 women-years' of use (that is, 100 women for one year, 50 women for two years, ten women for ten years).

One problem with this figure is that the longer the follow-up of participating women, the better the Pearl Index figure looks. This is because those who are going to become pregnant tend to do so early on – either because they take chances, misunderstand the method, are ambivalent about having children, or because the particular method under study fails to cover their biological circumstances.

The longer one follows up the women the lower the rate gets. Furthermore in initiating studies to measure effectiveness, if those who have been practising the method for several years are allowed to enrol, the apparent effectiveness will be much greater than if the study were limited to the new contraceptors. This is true even if you adjust for age, parity, and all the other demographic variables which we know will influence the Pearl Index.[1]

Robert Potter of Brown University, USA, comments: 'By allowing the successful contraceptors to contribute long-enough histories, a respectable Pearl Index pregnancy rate can be wrested from almost any sample.'[2]

PEARL INDEX FORMULA

pregnancy rate
expressed as $=$ $\dfrac{\text{no. of pregnancies}}{\text{no. of women-months of exposure}}$ $\times$ 1200 (or 1300 which relates to lunar months)
a percentage

To overcome weaknesses of the Pearl Index, other assessment methods have been devised, mainly aimed at taking account of the discontinuation rate as well as the pregnancy rate. Such methods are termed 'life table analyses' and are used more frequently in current reports.

The discontinuation rate gives some indication of whether side-effects are common, and whether couples find the method satisfactory to use.

Thorough assessment

In assessing the value of any fertility control method, careful examination of trial figures, teaching materials, teacher attitudes, the motivation of couples, acceptability, as well as any physical and psychological side-effects are important. Such thorough assessments are only just beginning.

Thus, for example, trial results of the Pill do not usually include a total failure rate (the oft-quoted one per cent failure rate of the Pill refers to the biological method failure rate). In studies which include those women who were unable or unwilling to tolerate the Pill and abandoned it as a means of contraception, the total pregnancy rate is as high as 20 per cent in a year.[3]

Tonga

One of the first published trials of the Ovulation Method was conducted on Tonga in the Pacific in 1970–72.[4]

Among 282 Tongan women who used the method for a total of 2503 months, one pregnancy resulted from an apparent failure of the method, and two pregnancies were classified as teaching-related failures.

A method-related pregnancy was recorded when the couple had understood and carried out the instructions faithfully. A teaching-related pregnancy was recorded when there was an error on the part of the couple which the teacher could explain to their satisfaction.

A further fifty women who consciously deviated from the guidelines became pregnant after having intercourse on a day when they recognized fertile mucus, and they therefore had no difficulty in realizing why pregnancy had occurred. Forty-nine of these women said that they intended to use the method after the birth of their babies.

In this trial, the method-related pregnancy rate (based on Pearl Index calculations) was 0.5 pregnancies per 100 women-years of use (that is, if 100 women used the method according to the guidelines, at most one pregnancy would occur in a year). The Pearl Index figure for total pregnancies was 25 per cent.

Sometimes it needs a pregnancy to prove to couples that the method works . . . Establishment of the method is accompanied by feelings of relief and freedom. Many women quickly determine to pass on the information about the method to other women, and in particular to instruct their daughters so that they, too, can space their families.
– M. C. Weissman, chief investigator, Tonga study.

Australia

Ball (1976)[5] studied 122 Ovulation Method users recruited from Natural Family Planning Centres throughout Australia. A total of 1626 cycles were investigated, with each woman averaging thirteen cycles of use of the method.

All participants had proven fertility – having carried at least one pregnancy to term – and all had observed at least one ovulatory cycle since the last birth.

The method-related pregnancy rate was 2.9 per cent (four pregnancies).

Examination of the pregnancies following apparent adherence to the guidelines indicated that the sperm must have survived five to six days in one case, six to seven days in two cases, and seven to eight days in the other.

A sperm survival time of up to five days is credible in the presence of adequate amounts of fertile mucus, but present scientific knowledge does not allow a clear statement about sperm viability for longer than this. Considerable doubt must be expressed about sperm survival for longer than five days when no fertile mucus is present.

What seems more likely is that the pregnancies did not result from the particular acts of intercourse specified, and that the method failure rate in this trial was even lower than the 2.9 per cent reported.

The teaching-related pregnancy rate was 5.9 per cent. This unusually high figure was thought to be due to misunderstanding of a recent innovation in the teaching.

The total pregnancy rate was 15.5 per cent (resulting from couples taking a chance, or deciding to exercise their second option of having a child).

Korea

This trial involved 2548 couples using the Ovulation Method for a total of 11 064 cycles.[6]

The method-related pregnancy rate was calculated at 1.7 per cent. The teaching-related pregnancy rate was 5.3 per cent, and a total pregnancy rate of 13.6 per cent was found using the Pearl formula (including the risk-takers and couples deciding to exercise the second option).

Eight further studies involving 2949 couples during four years show that the method is highly successful where couples follow the guidelines. These studies have yielded a constant total pregnancy rate of 11 per cent.

India – Tiruchirapalli[7]

One thousand couples participated in this trial during 1978 and 1979. Approximately two-thirds of the couples were

Christians, and the remainder were either Hindus (292 couples) or Muslims (26 couples). The aim of 187 of the couples was to achieve a pregnancy using the Ovulation Method. Forty-six per cent of couples did so (86 pregnancies). Among the remaining 813 couples who wished to avoid a pregnancy, three pregnancies occurred. Upon analysis, these were seen to be teaching-related pregnancies.

This trial is noteworthy because it contained a high proportion of breastfeeding mothers (195), and some women (13) who were approaching the menopause. Both groups found the method worked well. At the conclusion of the trial which lasted for one year, six couples had dropped out. The net cumulative continuation rate was thus 99.52 per cent.

Australia – Sydney[8]

The reported method-related pregnancy rate of 11.2 per cent, when compared with the 0 to 2.9 per cent method-related pregnancy rates of other trials points to inadequacies in teaching and assessment of pregnancies. This poor result was predicted after an examination of the teacher-training materials used in the trial.

Australia – Melbourne[9]

This study involved ninety-eight women who were judged to be approaching the menopause on the basis of hormonal studies, and who wished to find a natural solution to their family planning problems. The women ranged in age from thirty-eight to fifty-four years, and each was followed up during an average of three to four years. The total number of pregnancies was one, which occurred when a woman tested the guidelines and had intercourse on a day within the identified fertile phase.

The method-related pregnancy rate was zero, confirming that the pattern of the cervical mucus provides women who are approaching the menopause with a reliable means of assessing their current state of fertility or infertility. As for acceptability –

one woman required a hysterectomy when abnormalities were detected; no others discontinued.

Ireland – Dublin[10]

Can the method be used successfully after childbirth?

This study of fifty-five mothers with eighty experiences of breastfeeding who were using the Ovulation Method to identify infertility and fertility found that:

• All women identified the pattern of mucus leading to their first Peak of fertility after a time of prolonged infertility while breastfeeding. Eighty-four per cent said they found the identification 'easy'.

• Twenty-one per cent of women menstruated before the appearance of any fertile mucus, indicating a certainly infertile first cycle.

• Mothers who introduced solids after six months and who used the breast as a pacifier were likely to remain infertile for twelve months or longer.

This study demonstrates that during lactation, women can recognize signs of approaching fertility, no matter how long it is delayed. This information can be used to avoid or achieve a pregnancy.

USA – Los Angeles

This trial, conducted at the Cedars-Sinai Hospital in California and funded by the US Government Department of Health, Education and Welfare, aimed to compare the Ovulation Method with Sympto-Thermal methods of natural family planning.

The total pregnancy rate for the Ovulation Method was 24.8 per cent and for the Sympto-Thermal methods, 11.2 per cent.[11]

Although the pregnancies were not classified into those related to the method, to teaching or to a decision to have a child, it is known that the method-related pregnancy rate was low and comparable with that of other Ovulation Method trials.

The discontinuation rate for the Ovulation Method was exceedingly high (36.6 per cent) and this is at variance with other trials. Instability of relationships seems to have been responsible for the high drop-out rate. Barrier methods, which were said by the recruitment personnel to be admissible during the learning phase, produced confusion and further drop-outs.

USA[12]

Between 1975 and 1977, Dr Hanna Klaus conducted a trial involving six Ovulation Method centres and 1139 participating women. Of these 1090 wished to avoid pregnancy, 44 wanted to become pregnant and 5 women learned about the method while pregnant, intending to use it after delivery.

Amongst the 1090 women using the method to avoid pregnancy, the method-related pregnancy rate was one per cent. The total pregnancy rate, including those who did not follow the method guidelines, was 21 per cent.

At the end of two years, 56 per cent were continuing to use the method to avoid pregnancy, 4 per cent were now planning pregnancy, and 107 of those who had become pregnant (10 per cent) were planning to resume the use of the method following delivery.

World Health Organization trial[13]

This multi-centre clinical evaluation of the Ovulation Method is a project of the World Health Organization (WHO) programme of research, development and research training in human reproduction.

In August 1976, recruitment began with the aims of:
• Determining the percentage of women able to recognize changes in cervical mucus during the menstrual cycle
• Correlating the changes in the mucus with an objective marker of ovulation, namely levels of the hormone, progesterone
• Determining the effectiveness of the method.

In order to enable a cross-cultural assessment of the method, centres in New Zealand, Ireland, India, the Philippines and El Salvador were chosen. These centres had previous experience in the method, and qualified teachers were available. By June 1978, 875 women had joined the study. Special features of the study included:

• Selection of women who had not learned the method previously, and with proven fertility

• The inclusion of women with regular menstrual cycles only (lasting 23 to 35 days)

• Successful completion of a three-to-five-month training period before entering the main part of the effectiveness study

• Inclusion of women from both city and country areas at each centre.

Preliminary results[13, 14] indicate that:

• At least 90 per cent of women can produce a recognizable chart of their fertility after one teaching session. By the third teaching session, at least 94 per cent can recognize such a pattern.

• The method failure rate of this and similar studies is between one and three per cent.

• The total pregnancy rate is about 20 per cent. The vast majority of these pregnancies followed intercourse during the phase of recognized fertility. (The method-related pregnancy rate was 0.9 per cent for the three cycles of observation during the teaching phase, a period too short to make reliable judgements about overall method effectiveness. the teaching-related pregnancy rate was 5.3 per cent. Conscious departure from the method accounted for 12.9 per cent and unexplained, was 0.9 per cent.)

Conclusion

The trials demonstrate that the method is applicable in all phases of reproductive life, and in a wide range of social conditions.

The World Health Organization and other researchers have found that, biologically speaking, the method has a success rate of 97 to 99 per cent and that women are able to identify accurately and quickly the pattern of mucus that corresponds to fertility or infertility, as established by hormone investigations.

The vast majority of pregnancies that occur in the trials are not due to a failure of the method. Inadequate teaching has been a factor in some pregnancies. The cause is most often a decision to ignore the guidelines.

The Ovulation Method is an effective fertility regulation method if women are motivated to be aware of their own bodies, and then if they and their partners act in accordance with the sensations and observations of the mucus.

Essential to successful use of the method – either to avoid or achieve pregnancy – is a couple's concern for each other. The biological factor is near perfect, and provides a reliable foundation on which to base the human relationship.

Self test

1. How can the Billings Method be used to achieve a pregnancy?
2. How can the method be used to avoid a pregnancy?
3. Can the Billings Method be used when you are not ovulating?
4. Do all charts of the mucus look the same?
5. Will your own consecutive charts be similar?
6. What is meant by charting your normal cycle?
7. Is internal examination a useful method of mucus observation?
8. Describe the two major types of sensation you experience in a cycle.
9. Describe the fertile-type mucus.
10. Why should sexual intercourse be avoided during the first month of charting?
11. When do you make your mucus observations?
12. When do you record your observations?
13. What do you record on your chart?
14. How long does it take to establish a Basic Infertile Pattern in an unfamiliar situation such as when approaching the menopause?
15. What is the Peak mucus?
16. How is the Peak identified?
17. For how long after the Peak should intercourse be avoided?
18. How could genital contact without sexual intercourse during days of fertile-type mucus result in a pregnancy?

19. What is the Basic Infertile Pattern?

20. Are the days of menstruation available for sexual intercourse?

21. What time of day is available for intercourse during the Basic Infertile Pattern?

22. What may be the effect of stress on a woman's menstrual cycle?

Answers

1. By identifying the fertile days of the menstrual cycle, especially near the day of Peak mucus, and using these for sexual intercourse.

2. By identifying fertile days of the menstrual cycle and avoiding sexual intercourse and genital contact at these times.

3. Yes; the method is applicable to all circumstances of reproductive life. In the absence of ovulation, the method would indicate menstruation and an almost uninterrupted infertile phase.

4. No; because each woman's mucus pattern is individual to her, charts vary considerably.

5. Similar patterns *may* appear consecutively, although this is not necessarily the case.

6. Mucus observations are made by: awareness of sensations during normal activities; noticing visual characteristics of the mucus at the vaginal opening.

7. No; internal examination may cause confusion because the inside of the vagina is always moist. It may also cause infection or be culturally unacceptable.

8. Either a dry sensation; or a wet, damp or slippery, lubricative sensation.

9. It may be wet, clear, stretchy, stringy and possibly blood-stained. It has a lubricative sensation and has the consistency and appearance of raw egg-white. You may have very little mucus. You may not see it but will feel the lubrication.

10. This is necessary in order to obtain a clear picture of the

mucus, since seminal fluid or vaginal secretions may be lost from the vagina even on the day after intercourse. This could conceal the presence of fertile-type mucus.

11.   Throughout the day, in the course of normal activities.

12.   At the *end* of the day.

13.   All the relevant observations of the day *plus* the appropriate stamp, *plus* a description of the most fertile characteristics of the mucus.

14.   Two weeks observation is necessary.

15.   This occurs on the last day of the fertile-type mucus and occurs when fertility is maximal.

16.   It is identified retrospectively, on the following day when the pattern of infertile-type mucus or dry days begins to return.

17.   Three days.

18.   A drop of semen may escape from the penis, and the fluid may contain sperm cells which could fertilize an egg.

19.   Either dry days, and/or days of unchanging infertile-type mucus.

20.   No; because in a short cycle ovulation may occur before or immediately after bleeding is finished. Thus the fertile mucus may be concealed by the bleeding.

21.   Intercourse should be confined to the evenings if the aim is to avoid a pregnancy; this enables you to confirm that the Basic Infertile Pattern has been recognized on that day.

22.   Ovulation, and its mucus indications, may be delayed.

Teaching centres

AUSTRALIA	Vic.	Ovulation Method Centre 27 Alexandra Parade North Fitzroy, Melbourne Tel. 03 481-1722
	N.S.W.	Ovulation Method Centre 'The Cellar' 63A Carrington Road Waverley, Sydney
	A.C.T.	Ovulation Method Centre P.O. Box 167 Manuka, Canberra
	S.A.	W.O.O.M.B. – S.A. P.O. Box 258 Magill, Adelaide Tel. 08 794 494
	Qld.	Ovulation Method Centre Calvary Hospital Abbot Street Cairns
		Ovulation Method Centre 34 Hume Street Harlaxton Toowoomba
	W.A.	Ovulation Method Centre 19 Hebbard Street Samson, Perth

Tas. Ovulation Method Centre
10 Michael Street
West Launceston

N.T. Ovulation Method Centre
Sanderson Community
Health Centre
Darwin

BRITAIN National Association of
Ovulation Method Instructors
47 Heathhurst Road
Sanderstead
South Croydon, Surrey

CANADA Natural Family Planning
3050 Younge Street # 205
Toronto, Ontario

Billings Method Centre
Campus Ministry
Dalhousie University
Student Union Building
University Avenue
Halifax, Nova Scotia

Billings Method Centre
1506 Dansey Avenue
Coquitlam, B.C.

Billings Method Centre
C.P. 1091
Sherbrooke, P.Q.

CENTRAL Ovulation Method Centre
AMERICA 5A Ave, 10–38 Zona 1
Guatemala

COOK ISLANDS Ovulation Method Centre
St Joseph's School
Raratonga

FIJI   Responsible Parenthood Council
                        Box 5175
                        Raiwaqa

INDIA   Ovulation Method Centre
                        C.B.C.I. Centre
                        Ashok Place
                        New Delhi

IRELAND   Ovulation Method Advisory Service
                        19 Lower Mount Street
                        Dublin 2

                        NAOMI–OMAS Office
                        25 Grand Parade
                        Cork
                        Tel. 021–22213

ITALY   Billings Method Centre
                        Villa Maria
                        226 Via Appia Antica
                        Roma 00178

JAPAN   Ovulation Method Centre
                        3/8/37 Kengun
                        Kumanoto/Shi
                        Kumanoto/Ken, 862

KENYA   Ovulation Method Centre
                        Hughes Building
                        P.O. Box 48062
                        Nairobi, Kenya

KOREA   Ovulation Method Centre
                        St Columban's Hospital
                        Mokpa
                        Chollanando 680

MALAYSIA   Ovulation Method Centre
                    St Angela's School
                    P.O. Box 159
                    Seria, Brunei

NEW ZEALAND   Family Life Centre
                    36 Ihaka Street
                    Palmerston North

NIGERIA   Ovulation Method Centre
                    P.O. Box 20
                    Ondo

PAPUA   Ovulation Method Centre
NEW GUINEA   P.O. Box 5287
                    Erima,
                    Boroko

PHILIPPINES   Ovulation Method Centre
                    Family Life Education Office
                    Kamague
                    Iligan City

SINGAPORE   Ovulation Method Centre
                    Mt Alvernia Hospital
                    Thomson Rd
                    Singapore 20

SOUTH AFRICA   Ovulation Method Centre
                    St Joseph's Hospital
                    40 Park Drive
                    Port Elizabeth, 6001

TONGA   Ovulation Method Centre
                    P.O. Box 13
                    Nuku Alofa

URUGUAY

Ovulation Method Centre
Institute de Formacia
Familiar Social
Lavallega 2115
Montevideo

USA

Billings Ovulation Method Center
Department of Health and Hospitals
1400 W. Ninth Street
Los Angeles, California

Billings Method Center
Route 1, Box 366
Tchefuncta Country Club Estate
Covington, Louisiana

Natural Family Planning Center
c/ Dept of Obstetrics and
Gynecology
St Vincent's Hospital
Cnr 7th Ave and 11th St
New York

Natural Family Planning
Foundation
1511 K Street
N.W. Washington D.C.

Professor Thomas W. Hilgers
Department of Obstetrics and
Gynecology
Creighton University
Omaha, Nebraska

Twin Cities N.F.P. Centre
North Memorial Medical Centre
3220 Lowry Avenue
Minneapolis, Minnesota

References

Chapter 2 THE MUCUS DISCOVERY

1. W. T. Pommerenke, *American Journal of Obstetrics and Gynecology*, 52: 1023, 1946.
2. E. Rydberg, *Acta. Obstet. Gynec. Scand.*, 29(facs. 1): 127, 1948.
3. M. A. Breckenridge and W. T. Pommerenke, 'Analysis of carbohydrates in human cervical mucus', *Fertility and Sterility*, 2: 29, 1952.
4. M. R. Cohen, I. F. Stein and B. M. Kaye, *Fertility and Sterility*, 3: 202, 1952.
5. W. T. Smith, *The Pathology and Treatment of Leucorrhoea*, Churchill, London, 1855.
6. J. M. Sims, *British Medical Journal*, 2: 465–92, 1868.
7. M. Huhner, *Sterility in Male–Female and its Treatment*, Redman Co., New York, 1913.
8. J. Seguy and H. Simmonet, *Gynec. et Obstet.*, 28: 657, 1933.

Chapter 3 GETTING TO KNOW YOUR MENSTRUAL CYCLE

1. A. E. Treloar, R. E. Boynton, B. G. Behn, G. B. Borghild and B. W. Brown, 'Variation of the human menstrual cycle through reproductive life', *International Journal of Fertility*, 12: 77–126, 1970.

Chapter 4 THE KEY TO FERTILITY CONTROL – THE MUCUS

1. E. L. Billings, J. J. Billings, J. B. Brown and H. G. Burger, 'Symptoms and hormonal changes accompanying ovulation', *Lancet*, 1: 282–4, 1972.
2. C. G. Hartman, *Science and the Safe Period*, The Williams and Wilkins Co., Baltimore, 1962, pp.69–71.

Chapter 7 QUESTIONS OFTEN ASKED

1. Dr (Sr) Leonie McSweeney, Report to VIth International Institute of the Ovulation Method, Los Angeles, 1980.
2. T. W. Hilgers, Report to the VIth International Institute of the Ovulation Method, Los Angeles, 1980.
3. E. L. Billings, Study of Pre-Menopausal Women, Report to Workshop of the Ovulation Method, Sydney, 1973.
4. H. H. Mascarenhas, A. Lobo, A. S. Ramesch *et al.*, 'The use effectiveness of the Ovulation Method in India', *Indian Journal of Preventive and Social Medicine*, 10: 2, June 1979.
5. C. B. Haliburn, Report to VIth International Institute of the Ovulation Method, Los Angeles, 1980.
6. H. Klaus *et al.*, 'Use effectiveness and client satisfaction in six centres teaching the Billings Ovulation Method', *Contraception*, 19: 6, 613, 1979.

Chapter 8 LEARNING ABOUT FERTILITY IN ADOLESCENCE

1. J. G. Deaton and E. J. Pascoe, *The Book of Family Medical Questions*, Random House, New York, 1979, p.112.
2. *Handbook on sexually transmitted diseases*, National Health and Medical Research Council (Australia), April 1977.

Chapter 9 COMING OFF THE PILL

1. J. R. Evrard *et al.*, 'Amenorrhoea following oral contraception', *American Journal of Obstetrics and Gynecology*, 124: 88, 1976.
2. Editorial, 'Amenorrhoea after oral contraceptives', *British Medical Journal*, 18 September, 1976, pp.660–61.
3. US Food and Drug Administration, detailed patient labelling leaflet on contraception, April 1978.

Chapter 10 BREASTFEEDING AND THE BILLINGS METHOD

1. N. Leach, scientist and teacher, Ovulation Method Advisory Service, Dublin, Ireland, personal communication.
2. R. Short, director, Medical Research Council, Unit of Reproductive Biology, Edinburgh, personal communication.
3. J. B. Brown, Professor of Obstetrics and Gynaecology, University of Melbourne, Organon Lecture, Sydney, 1 September, 1978.
4. ibid.
5. ibid.
6. *Food and Nutrition and Reviews* (Aust.), 35: 3, 124, 1978.

Chapter 11   APPROACHING THE MENOPAUSE

1.   D. M. de Kretser and J. S. Jacobs, 'The endocrinologist's investigation of the infertile couple', *Medicine*, 9: 409–442, 1978.
2.   A. Rosenfield, 'Oral and intrauterine contraception: a 1978 risk assessment', *American Journal of Obstetrics and Gynecology*, 132: 92, 100, 1978.
3.   L. Dennerstein, G. Burrows, L. Cox and C. Wood, *Gynaecology, Sex and Psyche*, Melbourne University Press, Melbourne, 1978, p.167.
4.   E. L. Billings, Report to Workshop on the Ovulation Method, Sydney, 1973.
5.   H. G. Burger, 'Oestrogen replacement, a boon or a curse', *Australian Family Physician*, 6, 9 February 1977.
6.   C. B. Hammond, F. R. Jelovsek, K. L. Lee, W. T. Creasman and R. T. Parker, 'The effects of long-term oestrogen replacement therapy. II Neoplasia', *American Journal of Obstetrics and Gynecology*, 133, 537, 1979.
7.   H. Jick, R. N. Watkins *et al.*, 'Replacement estrogens and endometrial cancer', *New England Journal of Medicine*, 300, 218, 1979.
8.   J. G. Deaton and E. J. Pascoe, *The Book of Family Medical Questions*, Random House, New York, 1979, p.117.
9.   K. Little, *Bone Behaviour*, Academic Press, London and New York, 1973, pp.301–8.

Chapter 12   DIFFICULTIES IN CONCEIVING

1.   P. Walsh, 'A new cause of male infertility', *New England Journal of Medicine*, 300: 5, 253, February 1979.
2.   S. J. Behrman and R. W. Kistner, *Progress in Infertility*, Little Brown, Boston, 1975.
3.   R. J. Pepperell, J. B. Brown and J. H. Evans, 'Management of female infertility', *Medical Journal of Australia*, 2: 774–8, 1977.
4.   ibid.
5.   ibid.
6.   ibid.
7.   R. Newill, *Infertile Marriage*, Penguin Books, Harmondsworth, 1974, p.86.
8.   R. J. Pepperell *et al.*, op cit.
9.   Editorial, 'Pathogenesis of pelvic inflammatory disease', *British Medical Journal*, 16 June 1979.

10.   W. C. Scott, 'Pelvic abscess in association with intrauterine contraceptive device', *American Journal of Obstetrics and Gynecology*, 131: 149–56, 1978.

11.   M. A. Khatamee, 'T-Mycoplasma in abortion and infertility', *The Female Patient*, 109–12, October 1978.

Chapter 13   THE TECHNOLOGICAL APPROACH
TO CONTRACEPTION

1.   US Food and Drug Administration, detailed patient labelling leaflet on contraception, April 1978.

2.   A. Rosenfield, 'Oral and intrauterine contraception: a 1978 risk assessment', *American Journal of Obstetrics and Gynecology*, 132: 92, 1978.

3.   R. P. Shearman, 'Recent advances in contraception technology', *Medical Journal of Australia*, 2: 767–72, 1971.

4.   R. Doll, Lecture, Royal Melbourne Hospital, 12 December 1975.

5.   H. Carey, Professor of Obstetrics and Gynaecology, University of New South Wales, personal communication.

6.   US Food and Drug Administration leaflet, op. cit.

7.   *World Health*, World Health Organization issue on Research in Family Planning, August–September 1978, p.29.

8.   ibid.

9.   ibid.

10.   K. Little, *Bone Behaviour*, Academic Press, London and New York, 1973, pp.284–7.

11.   A. Rosenfield, op. cit., p.93.

12.   Editorial, 'Thrombo-embolism and oral contraceptives', *British Medical Journal*, 213, 19 February 1974.

13.   A. Rosenfield, op. cit., p.93.

14.   J. I. Mann, R. Doll, M. Thorogood *et al.*, 'Risk factors for myocardial infarction in young women', *British Journal of Preventive and Social Medicine*, 30: 94, 1976.

15.   A. Rosenfield, op. cit., p.96.

16.   Oral contraception study of the Royal College of General Practitioners, 'Mortality among oral contraceptive users', *Lancet*, ii: 727–31, 1977.

17.   J. N. Currie and J. J. Billings, 'Strokes and contraceptive medication', *Medical Journal of Australia*, 1: 58, 1980.

18.   Boston Collaborative Drug Surveillance Program, 'Oral con-

traceptives and venous thromboembolic disease, surgically confirmed gallbladder disease and breast tumours', *Lancet* i: 1399, 1973.

19.   E. Weisberg, 'Questions Women Ask About the Pill', *Australian Prescriber*, 2, 3, 56, 1978.

20.   US Center for Disease Control, 'Increased risk of hepatocellular adenoma in women with long-term use of oral contraception', *Morbidity and Mortality Weekly*, Rep. 26: 293, 1977.

21.   H. A. Edmondsen *et al.*, 'Liver adenomas associated with use of oral contraceptives', *New England Journal of Medicine*, 294, 470–72, 1976.

22.   US Food and Drug Administration leaflet, op. cit.

23.   *World Health*, op. cit.

24.   R. Buchanan, 'Breastfeeding. Aid to infant health and fertility control', Population Reports Series, *Journal of Family Planning Programs*, No. 4, July 1975.

25.   La Leche League International (Illinois), 'Breast-feeding and the oral contraceptive pill', Information Sheet, No. 18, 1975.

26.   A. Rosenfield, op. cit., p.96.

27.   E. Stern, A. B. Forsythe, L. Youkeles *et al.*, 'Steroid contraceptive use and cervical dysplasia: Increased risk of progression', *Science*, 196: 1460, 1977.

28.   US Food and Drug Administration leaflet, op. cit.

29.   'Oral contraception proceedings of seminar, Adelaide, Australia', supplement in *Australian Family Physician*, 8–11 March 1977.

30.   J. R. Evrard *et al.*, 'Amenorrhoea following oral contraception', *American Journal of Obstetrics and Gynecology*, 124: 88, 1976.

31.   US Food and Drug Administration leaflet, op. cit.

32.   E. Weisberg, op. cit., p.55.

33.   Editorial, 'Amenorrhoea after oral contraceptives', *British Medical Journal*, 660–61, 19 September 1976.

34.   H. I. Shapiro, *The Birth Control Book*, Avon, New York, 1978, pp.46–8.

35.   ibid., p.61.

36.   E. Weisberg, op. cit., p.57.

37.   F. J. Kane, 'Evaluation of emotional reactions to oral contraceptive use', *American Journal of Obstetrics and Gynecology*, 12, 6, 968–71, 1976.

38.   *World Health*, op. cit.

39.   US Food and Drug Administration leaflet, op. cit.

40.   R. P. Shearman, op. cit.

41.   A. Rosenfield, op. cit., p.100.

42.   H. I. Shapiro, op. cit., pp.83–4.

43.   A. Rosenfield, op. cit., p.101.

44.   Editorial; 'Contraceptive methods – risks and benefits', *British Medical Journal*, 22, 9 September 1978.

45.   A. K. Jain and B. Moots, 'Fecundability following discontinuation of IUD use among Taiwanese women', *Journal of Biosocial Science*, 9: 137, 1977.

46.   US Food and Drug Administration leaflet, op. cit.

47.   R. Shearman, op. cit.

48.   US Food and Drug Administration leaflet, op. cit.

49.   ibid.

50.   R. Shearman, op. cit.

51.   US Food and Drug Administration leaflet, op. cit.

52.   L. Darveen, 'Injectible contraception in rural Bangladesh', *Lancet*, 846–8, 5 November 1977.

53.   US Food and Drug Administration leaflet, op. cit.

54.   L. Dennerstein *et al.*, op. cit., p.172.

55.   ibid., p.167.

56.   ibid., p.168.

57.   P. Jouannet, 'Evolution of the properties of semen immediately following vasectomy', *Fertility and Sterility*, April 1978.

58.   R. W. M. Rees, 'Vasectomy: Problems of follow-up', *Proceedings of the Royal Society of Medicine*, 66: 52, 1973.

59.   R. P. Marwood and V. Beral, 'Disappearance of spermatozoa from the ejaculate after vasectomy', *British Medical Journal* 1: 87, 13, 1979.

60.   J. M. Bedford and G. Zelikowsky, 'Viability of spermatozoa in the human ejaculate after vasectomy', *Fertility and Sterility*, 32, 460, 1979.

61.   M. Briggs, World Health Organization consultant on contraception, *Australian* newspaper, 14 July 1979.

62.   M. Carruthers, Director of Clinical Laboratory Services, Maudsley Hospital and Institute of Psychiatry, London, *Sun* newspaper, Melbourne, 1 May 1979.

Chapter 14   NATURAL METHODS

1.   US Food and Drug Administration, detailed patient labelling leaflet on contraception, April 1978.

2.   H. Burger, 'The Ovulation Method of fertility regulation', *Modern Medicine in Australia*, 39, April 1978.

3. J. J. Billings, *The Ovulation Method*, Advocate Press, Melbourne, 1980.

4. H. Shapiro, *The Birth Control Book*, Avon, New York, 1978, p. 128.

5. ibid., p.131.

6. ibid., p.131.

7. J. A. Johnston, D. B. Roberts and R. B. Spencer, 'A survey evaluation of the efficacy and efficiency of Natural Family Planning services and methods in Australia', St Vincent's Hospital, Sydney, 1978, p.iii.

Chapter 15 SCIENTIFIC RESEARCH INTO THE METHOD

1. J. B. Brown, 'The scientific basis of the Ovulation Method', in J. J. Billings *et al.*, *Atlas of the Ovulation Method*, Advocate Press, 1980.

2. H. Burger, J. B. Brown and K. Catt, 'Relationship between plasma luteinising hormone and urinary estrogen excretion during the menstrual cycle', *Journal of Clinical Endocrinology*, 28, 1508–12, 1968.

3. E. L. Billings, J. J. Billings, J. B. Brown and H. G. Burger, 'Symptoms and hormonal changes accompanying ovulation', *Lancet* i: 282–4, 1972.

4. A. M. Flynn and S. S. Lynch, 'Cervical mucus and identification of the fertile phase of the menstrual cycle', *British Journal of Obstetrics and Gynaecology*, 83; 856, 1976.

5. J. H. Casey, 'Midcycle hormonal profiles, cervical mucus and ovulation', Paper presented at the international symposium on human ovulation. Wayne State University School of Medicine, April 1977.

6. S. Cortesi, Paper presented at Primo Corso Nationale sul Metodo della Ovulazione Billings, Rome, December 1979.

7. T. W. Hilgers, G. Abraham and D. Cavanagh, 'The Peak symptom and estimated time of ovulation', *Natural Family Planning*, Vol. 52, No. 5, November 1978.

8. R. J. Pepperell, J. B. Brown and J. H. Evans, 'Management of female infertility', *Medical Journal of Australia*, 2: 774–8, 1977.

9. E. Odeblad, A. Hoglund *et al.*, 'The dynamic mosaic model of the human ovulatory cervical mucus', Proc. Nord. Fert. Soc. Meeting, Umea, January 1978.

10. E. L. Billings, J. J. Billings, J. B. Brown and H. G. Burger, op. cit., 282–4.

11.   World Health Organization Colloquium, 'The Cervical Mucus in Human Reproduction', Geneva, 1972.

12.   T. W. Hilgers and A. M. Prebill, 'Vulva observations as an index of fertility/infertility', *American Journal of Obstetrics and Gynecology*, 53, 1, 575, January 1979.

13.   T. W. Hilgers *et al.*, op. cit.

14.   C. Hartman, *Science and the Safe Period*, Williams and Wilkins Co., Baltimore, 1962, p.60.

15.   T. W. Hilgers *et al.*, op. cit.

16.   E. Viergiver and W. T. Pommerenke, 'Measurement of the cyclic variations in the quantity of cervical mucus and its correlation with basal temperature', *American Journal of Obstetrics and Gynecology*, 48: 321–8, 1944.

Chapter 16   TRIALS OF THE METHOD

1.   Bernard G. Greenberg, 'Method Effectiveness Evaluation', *Natural Family Planning*, Human Life Foundation, 284, 1973.

2.   R. G. Potter, 'Application of life table techniques to measurements of contraceptive effectiveness', *Demography*, 3, 299, 1966.

3.   C. Tietze and S. Lewit, *Family Planning Perspectives*, 3, 53, 1971.

4.   M. C. Weissman, L. Foliaki, E. L. Billings and J. J. Billings, 'A trial of the Ovulation Method of family planning in Tonga', *Lancet*, 813–16, 14 October 1972.

5.   M. Ball, 'A prospective field trial of the Ovulation Method', *European Journal of Obstetrical and Gynaecological Reproductive Biology*, 6/2, 63–6, 1976.

6.   Kyo Sang Cho, Report to World Health Organization Conference, Geneva, February 1976.

7.   C. B. Haliburn, Report to VIth International Institute of the Ovulation Method, Los Angeles, 1980.

8.   J. A. Johnston, D. B. Roberts and R. B. Spencer, 'A survey evaluation of the efficacy and efficiency of Natural Family Planning services and methods in Australia', St Vincent's Hospital, Sydney, 1978.

9.   E. L. Billings, Report to Workshop on the Ovulation Method, Sydney, 1973.

10.   N. Leach, Ovulation Method Advisory Service, Dublin, personal communication.

11.   M. E. Wade *et al.*, 'A randomised prospective study of the use effectiveness of two methods of natural family planning: an interim report', *American Journal of Obstetrics and Gynecology*, 134, 628, 1979.

12. H. Klaus *et al.*, 'Use effectiveness and client satisfaction in six centres teaching the Billings Ovulation Method', *Contraception*, 19: 6, 613, 1979.

13. H. Burger, Proceedings of International Seminar on Natural Family Planning, Dublin, October 1979 (in press).

14. J. Spieler, Report to Primo Corso Nazionale sul Metodo della Ovulazione Billings, Rome, December 1979.

Glossary

ADHESION A fibrous band of tissue that abnormally binds or interconnects organs or other body parts.

AMENORRHOEA The prolonged absence of menstruation.

ANOVULAR CYCLE A cycle where ovulation does not occur.

ANTIBIOTIC A drug, for example, penicillin, that is used to treat diseases caused by bacteria.

ANTIBODY A protein produced by the body's immune (defence) system in response to an intruder. Antibodies serve to render intruders harmless.

ARTIFICIAL INSEMINATION The depositing of semen in the vagina by means other than sexual intercourse.

BACTERIA Single-celled organisms, some of which cause disease, while others are helpful to the body.

BASAL BODY TEMPERATURE (BBT) The lowest normal body temperature recorded under conditions of absolute rest; taken immediately after waking and before rising.

BASIC INFERTILE PATTERN (BIP) The pattern of cervical mucus indicating relative inactivity of the ovaries before a follicle begins to mature.

BILLINGS METHOD A technique of natural fertility control in which days of infertility, possible fertility, and maximal fertility are identified by a woman's observations of mucus at the vaginal opening.

CAUTERY See TUBAL CAUTERY.

CERVIX The lower part of the uterus (womb) that projects into the vagina.

CHANGE OF LIFE The menopausal years, during which reproductive function ceases.

CHROMOSOME One of the forty-six microscopic units within each cell that carries the genetic material responsible for inherited characteristics.

CLIMACTERIC   See CHANGE OF LIFE.

COLOSTRUM   The first milk from the mother's breasts.

COLPOSCOPY   The technique of viewing the cervix under magnification.

CONCEIVE   To become pregnant.

CONCEPTION   The fusion of the sperm and egg cells.

CONDOM   A sheath of rubber or plastic worn over the penis to prevent conception.

CORPUS LUTEUM   The yellow structure formed in the ovary after the release of an egg cell. If the egg is fertilized, the corpus luteum grows and produces hormones that support the pregnancy for several months. In the absence of fertilization, it degenerates.

CRYOSURGERY   Surgery involving freezing of diseased tissue without significantly harming normal adjacent structures.

CURETTAGE   The scraping out of the lining of the uterus with an instrument called a curette.

CYST   Any sac-like structure containing fluid or semi-solid material.

DANAZOL   A synthetic medication similar in structure to the male hormone, testosterone, used for the treatment of endometriosis.

DEPO-PROVERA   A synthetic progesterone-like hormone used as a contraceptive.

DIAPHRAGM   A rubber, dome-shaped device worn over the cervix during intercourse to prevent conception.

DIATHERMY   A technique in which local heat is produced in the body tissues below the surface.

DILATATION AND CURETTAGE (D AND C)   A surgical procedure in which the cervix is gradually opened with instruments called dilators. Tissue is then removed from the surface of the endometrium and cervix with a curette.

DIXIRIT   A non-hormonal medication used to treat hot flushes (flashes).

DOUCHE   A substance flushed through the vagina.

DYSPAREUNIA   Painful or difficult intercourse.

EARLY DAY RULES   The Billings Method guidelines for avoiding a pregnancy in the days before fertile-type mucus occurs.

ECTOPIC PREGNANCY   A pregnancy that develops outside the normal location within the uterus. Ectopic pregnancies usually occur in the Fallopian tubes.

EGG CELL (OVUM)   The female cell that on fusion with a sperm cell can develop into a new individual.

EJACULATION   Discharge of semen from the penis.

EMBRYO   The initial stages in the formation of a baby in the uterus.

ENDOCRINOLOGIST   A doctor who specializes in the function of hormones.

ENDOMETRIOSIS   A condition caused by the presence of pieces of endometrium in areas other than the normal location within the uterus.

ENDOMETRIUM   The inner lining of the uterus.

ESTROGEN   See OESTROGEN.

ETHYNYL OESTRADIOL   A form of oestrogen that is effective in producing cervical mucus with fertile characteristics.

FALLOPIAN TUBES   The muscular tubes (two) along which the egg travels from the ovary to the uterus, and in which the egg is fertilized.

FERNING   The tendency of cervical mucus to form a fern-like pattern when dried on a glass slide.

FERTILE DAYS   The days of the menstrual cycle during which intercourse may result in a pregnancy.

FERTILE-TYPE MUCUS   Mucus from the cervix which is produced close to the time of ovulation. It has a slippery, lubricative sensation, tends to form strings, and resembles raw egg-white.

FERTILIZATION   The fusion of an egg and a sperm.

FERTILITY   The ability to reproduce.

FERTILITY DRUGS   A group of natural and synthetic substances capable of enabling some women to conceive.

FIBROIDS   Growth of muscle in the wall of the uterus.

FLUSHES (FLASHES)   See HOT FLUSHES.

FOETUS   The developing baby within the uterus.

FOLLICLE   A small fluid-filled structure within the ovary that contains the developing egg. At ovulation, the egg is released when the follicle breaks through the surface of the ovary.

FOLLICLE STIMULATING HORMONE (FSH)   The hormone produced by the pituitary gland that stimulates the ovaries to produce mature egg cells and oestrogen hormone.

GENETIC   Having to do with hereditary characteristics.

GENITAL   Having reference to the organs of reproduction.

GENITAL CONTACT   Contact of the penis with the vaginal opening, or tissues around it.

GONORRHOEA   A highly contagious venereal disease.

GYNAECOLOGIST   A doctor who specializes in the treatment and management of problems affecting the female reproductive system.

HAEMORRHAGE Excessively heavy bleeding.

HORMONE A chemical substance produced within the body which stimulates or affects other organs or body parts.

HOT FLUSHES Sudden flushing of the skin accompanied by perspiration and a feeling of intense heat.

HUHNER'S TEST Examination of the cervical mucus shortly after intercourse, to determine how receptive it is to sperm.

HYPOTHALAMUS A major control centre of the body, situated at the base of the brain, and interacting with the pituitary gland.

HYSTERECTOMY The surgical removal of the uterus and cervix.

HYSTEROSALPINGOGRAM An X-ray taken after a special dye is injected through the cervix. It produces an image of the inside of the uterus and the Fallopian tubes.

IMPLANTATION The embedding of the fertilized egg in the lining of the uterus.

IMPOTENCE The inability to obtain or maintain an erection of the penis.

INCOMPETENT CERVIX A cervix that is too weak to carry the weight of a growing pregnancy.

INFERTILE-TYPE MUCUS Mucus from the cervix that is flaky, crumbly, and opaque, and that forms a barrier to sperm cells.

INFERTILITY Temporary or permanent inability to conceive or reproduce.

INTERCOURSE Sexual relations involving the insertion of the penis into the vagina, with the release of sperm.

INTRAUTERINE DEVICE (IUD) Any device placed within the uterus for the purpose of avoiding a pregnancy.

LACTATION The production of milk by the breasts.

LAPAROSCOPY A procedure in which the inside of the abdomen, and particularly the ovaries, is examined using an instrument like a thin telescope (called a laparoscope).

LAPAROTOMY The surgical operation of opening the abdomen.

LIBIDO Sex drive; the desire for sexual intercourse.

LOCHIA The discharge from the uterus and vagina during the first few weeks after giving birth.

LUTEINIZING HORMONE (LH) A hormone from the pituitary gland in the brain that stimulates rupture of the follicle and ovulation.

MASTURBATE To obtain a sexual orgasm by self-manipulation of the genital organs.

MEMBRANE Moist layer of cells that lines body cavities and passageways.

MENARCHE The age at which menstruation begins.

MENOPAUSE The permanent cessation of menstruation.

MENSTRUAL CYCLE The time interval from the beginning of one menstrual cycle to the beginning of the next. During the cycle the endometrium develops, regresses, and is shed.

MENSTRUATION The period of bleeding from the uterus that occurs approximately monthly.

MINI PILL A type of birth control Pill that contains a progestogen but no oestrogen.

MUCUS, CERVICAL The secretion from the lining cells of the cervix.

OBSTETRICIAN A doctor who supervises pregnancy and childbirth.

OESTRADIOL A type of oestrogen.

OESTROGEN A hormone produced mainly in the ovaries that is responsible for female sexual characteristics and plays an important role in ovulation.

OSTEOPOROSIS The loss of calcium and other substances from bone, leading to its softening and weakening.

OVARIAN CYCLE A cyclic series of events occurring in the ovary during which an egg cell matures and is released.

OVARY The female sex organ in which egg cells mature and hormones are produced which influence the release of the egg cells.

OVULATION The release of an egg from the ovary.

OVULATION METHOD (BILLINGS METHOD) A technique of natural fertility control in which days of infertility, possible fertility, and maximum fertility are identified by a woman's observations of mucus at the vaginal opening.

OVUM See EGG CELL.

PEAK DAY The last day of fertile mucus characteristics in a menstrual cycle. It correlates closely with the time of ovulation.

PEAK RULE The Billings Method guidelines applying to the fertile days of the menstrual cycle.

PEARL INDEX A statistical measurement relating to pregnancies occurring among a trial group.

PELVIC INFLAMMATORY DISEASE (PID) Inflammation and/or infection involving the internal female reproductive organs. Commonly used to describe any acute, recurrent, or chronic infection of the Fallopian tubes and/or ovaries.

PENETRATION The insertion of the penis into the vagina.

PENIS The male organ inserted into the vagina during intercourse.

PERFORATED UTERUS A uterus in which the wall has been pierced, often inadvertently.

PITUITARY GLAND The gland at the base of the brain that produces many important hormones, including those essential for reproduction.

POLYCYSTIC OVARIES A condition in which the ovaries are studded with many small cysts.

POLYP A small growth, shaped like a tear-drop, often found in the cervix or endometrium.

POSTCOITAL TEST See HUHNER'S TEST.

PROGESTERONE The female hormone produced by the corpus luteum as a result of ovulation. It supports the developing pregnancy.

PROGESTOGEN A synthetic drug which has similar actions to progesterone.

PROLACTIN A hormone from the pituitary gland which stimulates breast milk production.

PROSTAGLANDINS Naturally occurring substances capable of stimulating the muscular contractions of the uterus.

PUBERTY The time of life in boys and girls when the reproductive organs become functional.

SEMEN The fluid ejaculated by a man during intercourse or masturbation; contains sperm.

SPERM The male reproductive cell which on fusing with an egg cell forms a new individual.

SPERMICIDAL Destructive to sperm.

SPERMICIDES Vaginal creams, foams, jellies, or suppositories that can immobilize or destroy sperm.

STERILIZATION A procedure to render an individual permanently unable to reproduce.

STERILITY The inability to conceive.

TESTES (TESTICLES) Male sex organs in which sperm and the hormone testosterone are produced.

THROMBOSIS A condition in which a plug or clot of blood partly or completely blocks a blood vessel.

TUBAL CAUTERY The sealing of the Fallopian tubes by burning, rendering them impassable to sperm and egg cells; a form of sterilization.

TUBAL LIGATION Surgical sterilization by tying a surgical string around a segment of the Fallopian tubes, thus preventing the egg and sperm from meeting.

TUBAL PREGNANCY   An ectopic pregnancy occurring in a Fallopian tube.

ULTRASOUND   A diagnostic technique which uses sound waves to produce an image of internal body structures.

UTERUS (WOMB)   The hollow muscular organ of reproduction in which the fertilized egg implants and develops.

VAGINA   The female organ or passage into which sperm are released during intercourse.

VAGINISMUS   A painful spasm of the vagina which prevents penetration by the penis.

VASECTOMY   A surgical sterilization procedure in which the vas deferens (the tube that carries sperm from the testes) is cut, and the ends separated, so that sperm can no longer pass through.

VENEREAL DISEASE (VD)   Any infection that is transmitted mainly by sexual intercourse.

WITHDRAWAL (COITUS INTERRUPTUS)   Sexual intercourse in which the penis is withdrawn and semen discharged outside the vagina.

WITHDRAWAL BLEEDING   The first bleeding after coming off the Pill.

ZYGOTE   The fertilized egg.

Index

Personal Record Chart

	1	2	3	4	5	6	7	8	9	10	11	12	13	14	15	16	17	18	19	20	21	22	23	24	25	26	27	28	29	30	31	32	33	34	35
Date / /																																			
Mucus																																			
Date / /																																			
Mucus																																			
Date / /																																			
Mucus																																			
Date / /																																			
Mucus																																			
Date / /																																			
Mucus																																			

More about Penguins and Pelicans

For further information about books available from Penguins please write to Dept EP, Penguin Books Ltd, Harmondsworth, Middlesex U B7 0DA.

In the U.S.A.: For a complete list of books available from Penguins in the United States write to Dept CS, Penguin Books, 625 Madison Avenue, New York, New York 10022.

In Canada: For a complete list of books available from Penguins in Canada write to Penguin Books Canada Ltd, 2801 John Street, Markham, Ontario L3R 1B4.

In Australia: For a complete list of books available from Penguins in Australia write to the Marketing Department, Penguin Books Australia Ltd, P.O. Box 257, Ringwood, Victoria 3134.

In New Zealand: For a complete list of books available from Penguins in New Zealand write to the Marketing Department, Penguin Books (N.Z.) Ltd, P.O. Box 4019, Auckland 10.